IMAGES
of America

SOUTH SHORE HOSPITAL

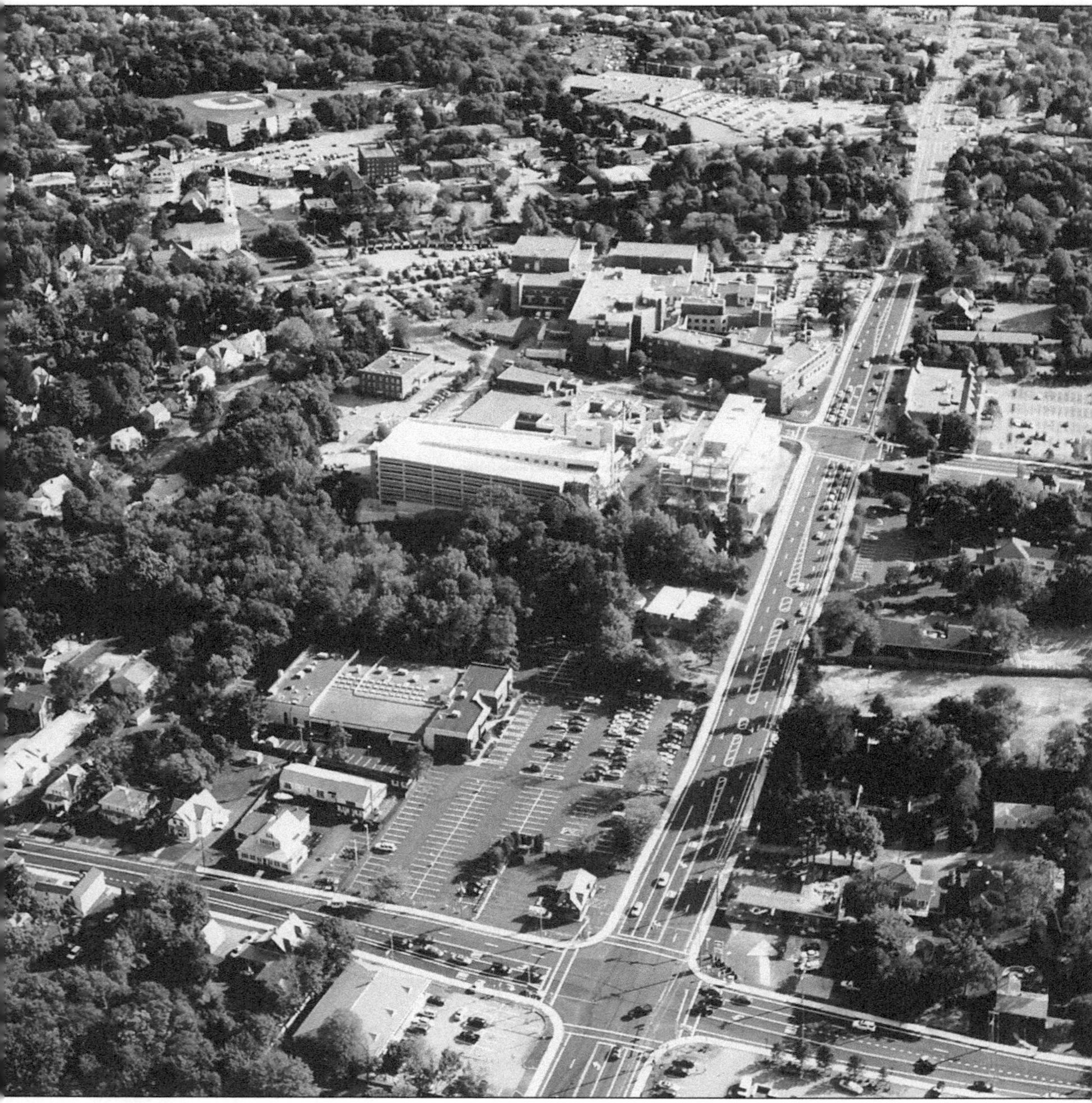

This aerial photograph looking south along Main Street (Route 18) shows the hospital campus in South Weymouth, Massachusetts. (Courtesy of South Shore Hospital.)

ON THE COVER: Sally Hurst (left) and Ann Campbell, residents of Weymouth, showed support for Weymouth Hospital (now South Shore Hospital) during World War II by donating fruits and vegetables from their victory garden on Central Street. These were used for patient meals. (Photograph by William Rittase, courtesy of South Shore Hospital.)

IMAGES
of America

SOUTH SHORE HOSPITAL

Richard Aubut and Myrna Walsh

ARCADIA
PUBLISHING

ISBN 978-1-5316-5083-4

Published by Arcadia Publishing
Charleston, South Carolina

Library of Congress Control Number: 2011934179

For all general information, please contact Arcadia Publishing:
Telephone 843-853-2070
Fax 843-853-0044
E-mail sales@arcadiapublishing.com
For customer service and orders:
Toll-Free 1-888-313-2665

Visit us on the Internet at www.arcadiapublishing.com

To South Shore Hospital's family—physicians, nurses, other caregivers, all staff, and volunteers devoted to healing, caring, and comforting patients and families.

Contents

ACKNOWLEDGMENTS

We thank all contributors to this history: Karen Baker, Georgia Buchanan, Judith Carron, Jane Cavanaugh, Camille Constantino, Patricia Coyte, Frances DeLorenzo, Katrina Dwyer, Roxanne Desmaris, Elizabeth Ezekiel, Carol Green, Ben Johnson, Lucy Kalaijian, Constance Libardoni, Elizabeth Lynch, Helen Lynch, Patrice Lynch Perrotta, Sally Sullivan, and Barbara Tilden. Rose DiPietro and Timothy Quigley made this history possible, and Paul Taylor was editor and head coach.

Unless otherwise indicated, all photographs appear courtesy of South Shore Hospital.

INTRODUCTION

At first it was personal. Dr. George F. Emerson steadied his wife as the labor contraction rolled through her body. She shivered from exhaustion and the bitter cold. Complications made the delivery difficult. He waited while the contraction subsided and gently helped her onto the streetcar, then the most practical way to travel to Boston hospitals. The ruts and bumps on the road made the trip by automobile precarious.

As he comforted his wife, he vowed to help women get better care close to home. The birth of the Emerson child in 1921 was the genesis that led to a progressive and innovative hospital serving a large region.

Some Boston doctors considered Emerson foolhardy, but he persisted. He reminded them of another patient with a ruptured appendix tied to a stretcher and sent to a Boston hospital in a train baggage car. This indignity and others sparked a quest for a new hospital.

The founders were men of courage and bold vision. They insisted that their new hospital be self-supporting and that no patient be turned away for inability to pay. The hospital never wavered from these standards despite financial hardship and overwhelming charity care. The more timid might have tried to replicate the so-called cottage hospital model of no more than 25 beds staffed with only general practitioners. The town's first cottage hospital on East Street, which was managed by the Weymouth Hospital Association, had closed several years earlier. These men, all successful community leaders like Emerson, were confident they could turn a mansion into a hospital. They boldly expanded, borrowed when necessary, and made enlightened decisions, often without a financial safety net.

The board created and supported the Guarantee Fund to assure the hospital's financial health. In 1933, the midst of the Depression, the staff voluntarily took pay cuts to continue charitable care. Board president W. Carleton Barnes proudly wrote, "During this fourth consecutive year of general financial and economic distress and disaster, our institution has carried on its work of caring for the sick and the injured with undiminished energy and activity."

The hospital faced continued financial hardships: a default by a major health insurer, World War II, the baby boom, conflicting signals from Washington, a shortage of nurses and physicians, an overabundance of patients, unpaid hospital bills, and uncertain reimbursement from Medicare and Medicaid. Through it all, the leaders and staff persevered and prevailed.

The founders also insisted on compassion. They created a cultural imperative of caring. The first bylaws called for a visiting committee of 12 members (no less than half were "ladies"). They had to visit the hospital weekly and report anything needing rectification. They provided flowers, food, and other amenities "so necessary in maintaining the atmosphere in an institution of this kind."

Among its early pioneering initiatives, Weymouth Hospital (now South Shore Hospital) became the first New England hospital to institute group hospitalization and insurance, known as the Weymouth Hospital Service Plan. The hospital was the first private organization in the nation to receive funding from the Public Works Administration (PWA), which purchased $60,000 of the hospital's four-percent bonds in 1934. Hospital president W. Carleton Barnes noted that the funding was given in recognition of the hospital's "highest grade and of great service to the community" and "our splendid record of progress."

South Shore Hospital was one of the first to offer 24-hour emergency room coverage and day surgery in a community hospital. It introduced advanced care for emergency, maternity, pediatric, surgical, cardiac, stroke, and cancer to the region.

The founders' values of personal responsibility, fiscal prudence, and compassion are now embedded into the hospital's culture and expressed thousands of times every day. They are codified in the hospital's values statement: "We care for our patients as we would our loved ones: with expertise, compassion, and respect. We personify initiative, innovation, and tenacity in addressing community health care priorities. We foster an environment that celebrates diversity, rewards excellence and added value, and encourages good citizenship. We work cooperatively with our colleagues and our community to advance the region's well-being. We exhibit leadership on critical issues, in ways worthy of public confidence. We demonstrate accountability, integrity, and resourcefulness in our financial stewardship."

These values are a touchstone that helped transform the hospital into a preeminent facility that combines the personal care of a community hospital with the medical expertise typically found in academic medical centers.

Dr. Arthur Sullivan, whose father was on the first medical staff, recalled care in 1922: "It was the age of the little black bag and house calls. This was before the days of antibiotics and modern medications. Treatment was basically to provide symptomatic relief and a generous application of reassurance."

In less than 100 years and from a 20-bed, converted pre–Civil War mansion, it became the hospital of superlatives. It is the largest provider of emergency, acute, outpatient, home health, and hospice care in southeastern Massachusetts, with a budget of $450 million. It is one of the largest non-government employers in southeastern Massachusetts. It operates one of the largest emergency and maternity services in the commonwealth. South Shore Visiting Nurses, the hospital's home-care division, is the state's fourth largest provider of home-care services.

The quality of care has been a hallmark from the earliest days. The hospital repeatedly earned the highest recognition for the quality of its care. The Commission on Trauma of the American College of Surgeons verified that the hospital met the standards of a Level II trauma center. The American Stroke Association recognized the staff's expertise in preventing and treating strokes. The Massachusetts Department of Public Health formally recognized South Shore Hospital as a Level III maternal and newborn program, the first and only community hospital in the commonwealth with this designation. As a Magnet hospital, its nursing program is ranked in the top seven percent in the nation.

From that start grew an extraordinary hospital. This history describes the remarkable journey that began at a Weymouth streetcar stop.

One

Weymouth Needs It

Cottage Hospital to Medical Center

George Benedict (board president in 1955) wrote, "Our building may look like just a pile of bricks to the passing motorist, but to the 6,800 patients of our last fiscal year, they have meant a place for the best in medical and surgical care, administered by a staff of men and women who serve not only with skill, but also with kindness, loyalty, and devotion."

The history of South Shore Hospital should begin with its brick-and-mortar exoskeleton, the most public indicator of its growth.

Using language ringing of manifest destiny, the founders created a prospectus for raising funds. They wrote, "We heartily endorse the Weymouth Hospital. . . . A very real need of a hospital in Weymouth has been recognized for many years, and the opportunity is now presented to meet that need in a most satisfactory manner. We urge all the people of Weymouth to assist to the fullest possible extent in the establishing of and supporting this Hospital. . . . Weymouth needs it and Weymouth can and will maintain it."

The founders moved with characteristic purpose. Only seven months passed between purchasing the H.B. Reed Mansion and its opening as Weymouth Hospital. Over 90 years, the hospital's leadership built, expanded, or renovated 15 buildings—not counting nurses' dormitories, power plants, garages, and satellite offices.

It began on May 21, 1922, an unseasonably warm day, with band music, cookies, and a speech by Gov. Channing H. Cox.

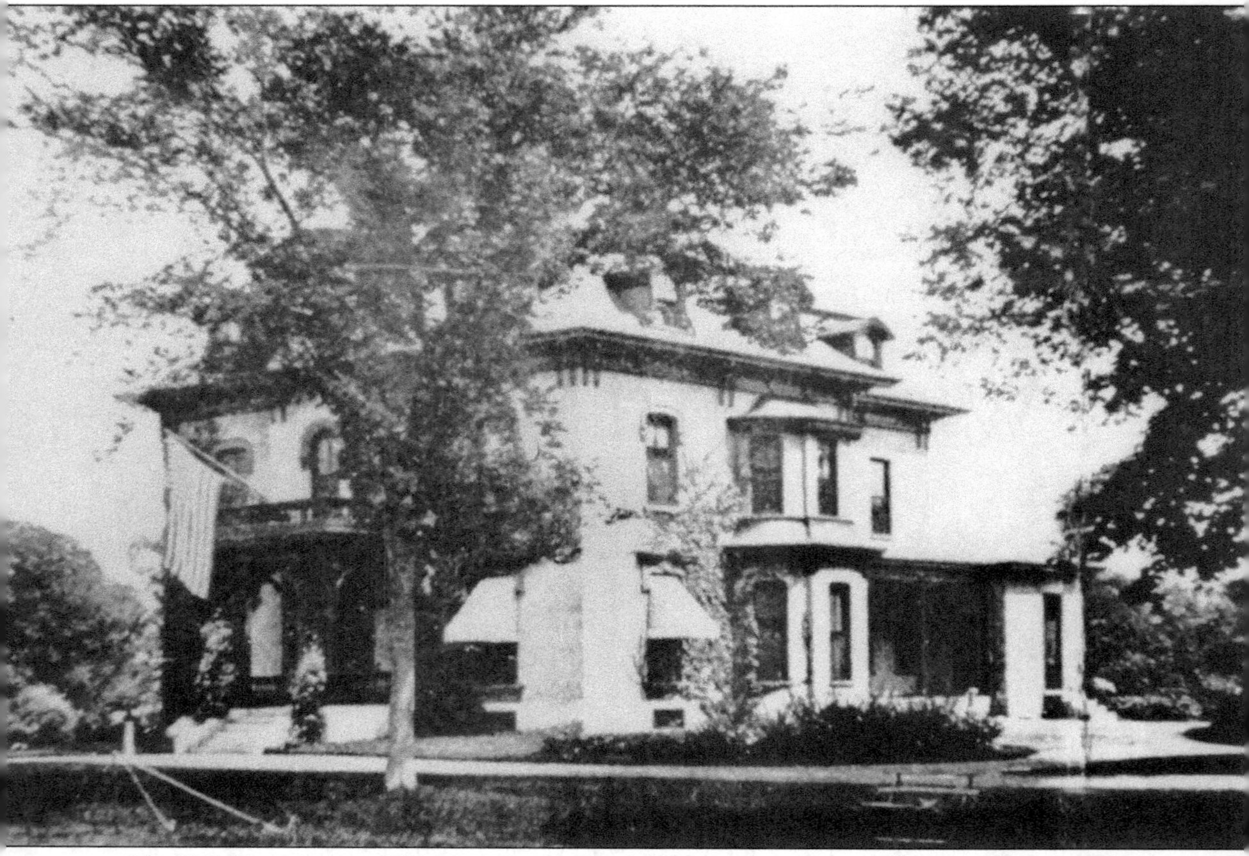

The H.B. Reed estate at 564 Main Street, South Weymouth, was centrally located at the corner of Columbian and Main Streets. The three-story brick house and stable was on three and a half well-landscaped acres atop a winding driveway. A fundraising prospectus stated, "The property furnishes an ideal location for hospital purposes, well adapted, with its pleasant and attractive surrounding, to materially aid in the convalescence of its patients. . . . The interior of the building requires no further alteration to properly accommodate from seventeen to twenty patients, on the first two floors." There were rooms for offices, a darkroom for developing X-ray film, and dining for nurses. In the basement near the coal box was ample space for storing vegetables. Heated by hot air, the Reed Mansion also included two plumbing systems and a ventilating system from each room to the roof. It was expected that additional patient rooms could be added in the attic.

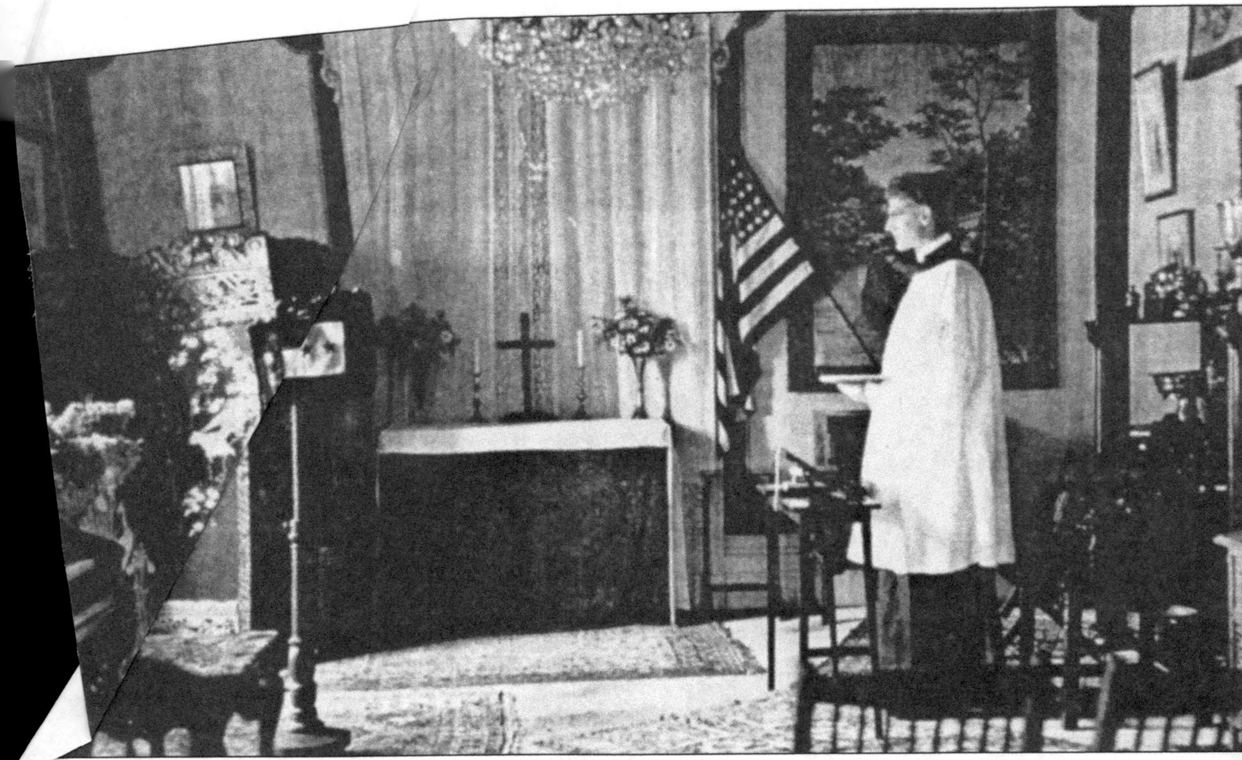

The mansion was originally built by Albert Tirrell prior to the Civil War. He sold it to H.B. Reed, a shoe manufacturer in South Weymouth and the first president of South Weymouth Savings Bank (now South Shore Savings Bank). Reed later sold the property to Col. Daniel Cornman. On Christmas Day 1915, the Cornmans hosted the first gathering of the Episcopal Church of the Holy Nativity in their drawing room. In this photograph, Rev. Robert Pierce Casey prepares for the service. The great crystal chandelier was later removed and the living room converted into an eight-bed ward. Neighbor and one of the original trustees, Alonzo Newbert bought the house, stable, and property from Cornman's estate for $1 and back taxes. Newbert then sold the buildings and property to Weymouth Hospital for $14,000. He dated the six-percent mortgage six months ahead, thereby donating six month's interest. After his death, his wife extended the mortgage on the remaining $4,000 from 1932 to 1935.

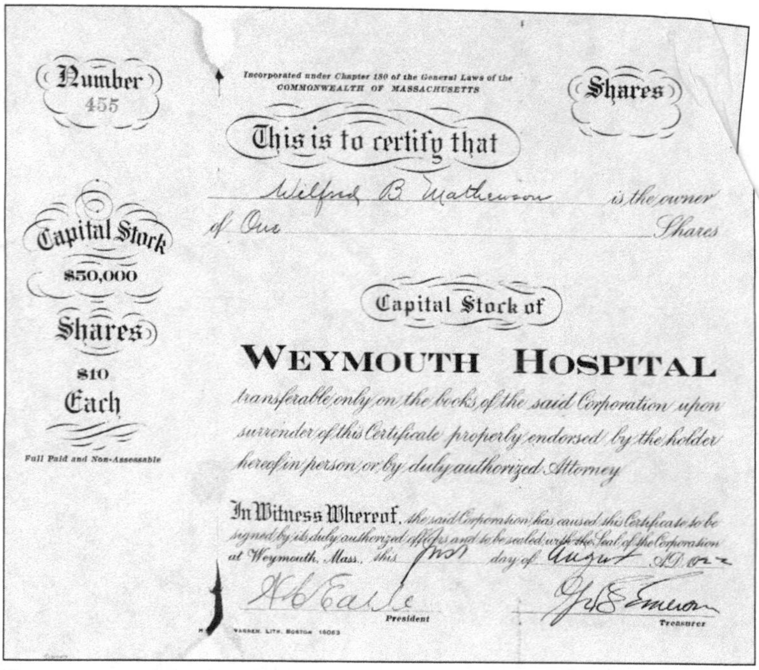

Number 455

Incorporated under Chapter 180 of the General Laws of the COMMONWEALTH OF MASSACHUSETTS

Shares

This is to certify that Wilfred B. Matherson is the owner of One Shares

Capital Stock $50,000

Shares $10 Each

Full Paid and Non-Assessable

Capital Stock of

WEYMOUTH HOSPITAL

transferable only on the books of the said Corporation upon surrender of this Certificate properly endorsed by the holder hereof in person or by duly authorized Attorney

In Witness Whereof, the said Corporation has caused this Certificate to be signed by its duly authorized officers and to be sealed with the Seal of the Corporation at Weymouth, Mass., this first day of August A.D. 1922

President

Treasurer

Wagner Lith. Boston 16063

To renovate the Reed Mansion, buy equipment, and pay the mortgage, hospital trustees issued 4,000 shares of "common stock" at a c value of $10. The likcates looked it wa stock, but decadermined not-for-pr that as a the hospitharity, legally own community, a e "stock certifica were actually jus clever thank-yous for philanthropy. Their only value is as historical artifacts.

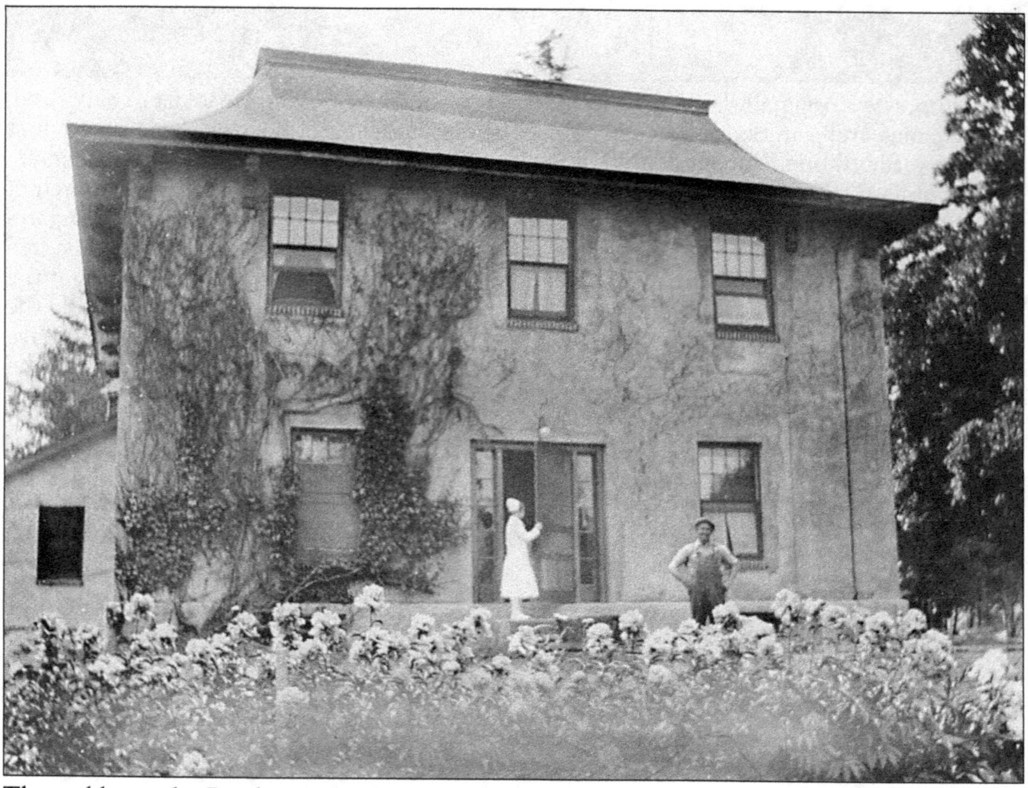

The stable on the Reed property was converted into a nurses' home for $11,000 in 1924. The nursing school opened with seven student nurses in September 1925 but lasted only a few years. The nurses' home was later replaced with a three-story dormitory at the corner of Main and Columbian Streets.

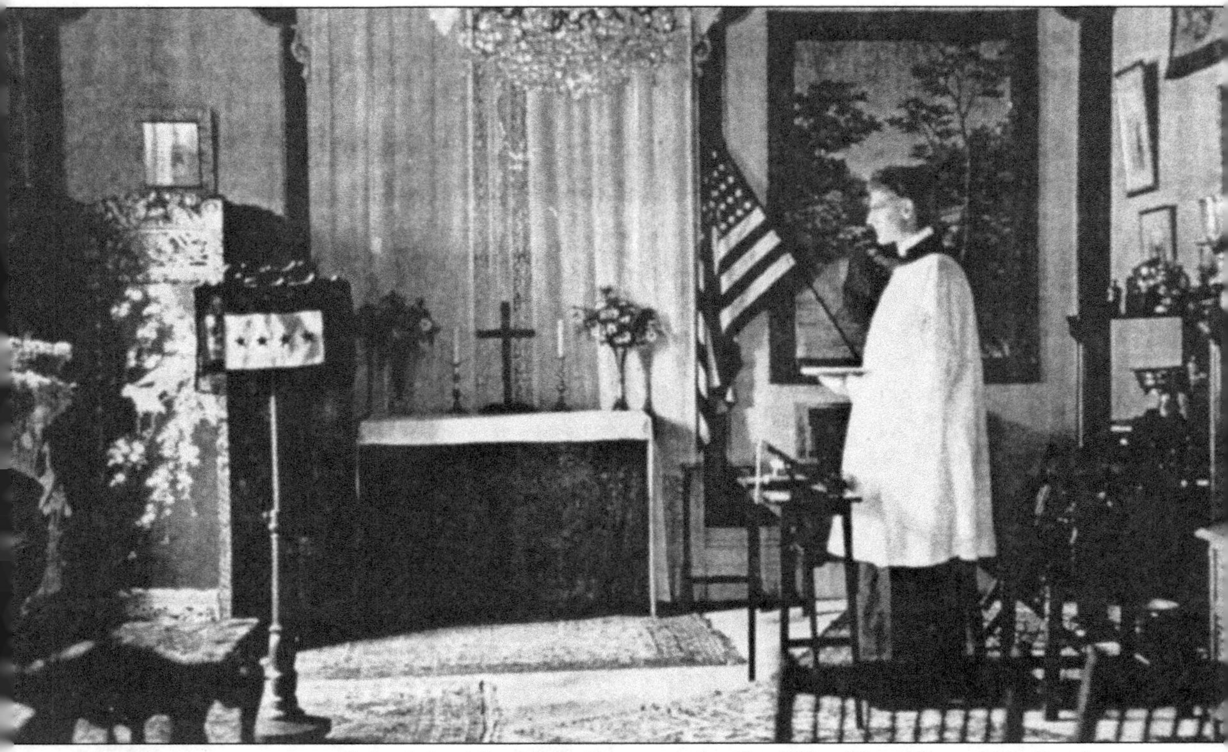

The mansion was originally built by Albert Tirrell prior to the Civil War. He sold it to H.B. Reed, a shoe manufacturer in South Weymouth and the first president of South Weymouth Savings Bank (now South Shore Savings Bank). Reed later sold the property to Col. Daniel Cornman. On Christmas Day 1915, the Cornmans hosted the first gathering of the Episcopal Church of the Holy Nativity in their drawing room. In this photograph, Rev. Robert Pierce Casey prepares for the service. The great crystal chandelier was later removed and the living room converted into an eight-bed ward. Neighbor and one of the original trustees, Alonzo Newbert bought the house, stable, and property from Cornman's estate for $1 and back taxes. Newbert then sold the buildings and property to Weymouth Hospital for $14,000. He dated the six-percent mortgage six months ahead, thereby donating six month's interest. After his death, his wife extended the mortgage on the remaining $4,000 from 1932 to 1935.

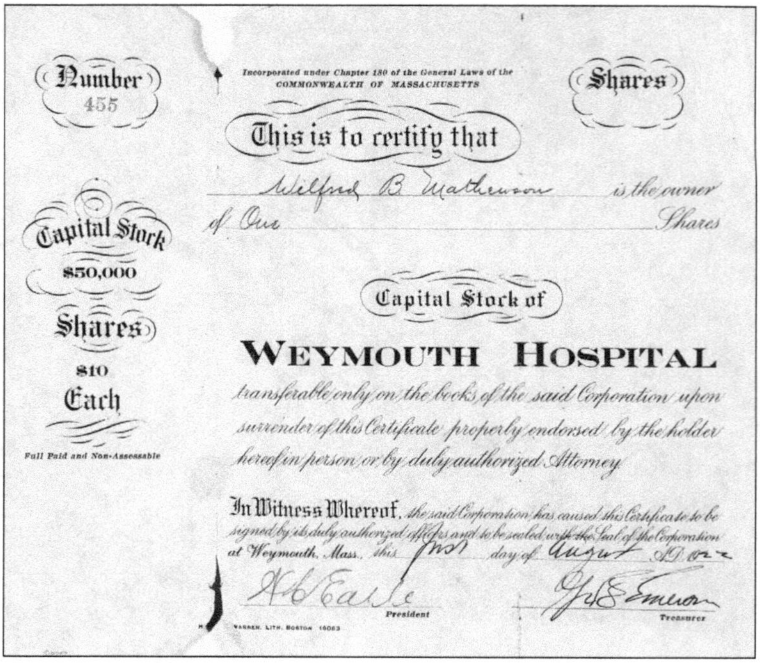

Number 455

Incorporated under Chapter 180 of the General Laws of the COMMONWEALTH OF MASSACHUSETTS

Shares

This is to certify that

Wilfred B. Mathewson is the owner of One Shares

Capital Stock $50,000

Shares $10 Each

Full Paid and Non-Assessable

Capital Stock of

WEYMOUTH HOSPITAL

transferable only on the books of the said Corporation upon surrender of this Certificate properly endorsed by the holder hereof in person or by duly authorized Attorney.

In Witness Whereof, the said Corporation has caused this Certificate to be signed by its duly authorized officers and to be sealed with the Seal of the Corporation at Weymouth, Mass. this first day of August A.D.

President

Treasurer

To renovate the Reed Mansion, buy equipment, and pay the mortgage, hospital trustees issued 4,000 shares of "common stock" at a par value of $10. The certificates looked like real stock, but it was determined decades later that as a not-for-profit charity, the hospital was legally owned by the community, and the "stock certificates" were actually just clever thank-yous for philanthropy. Their only value is as historical artifacts.

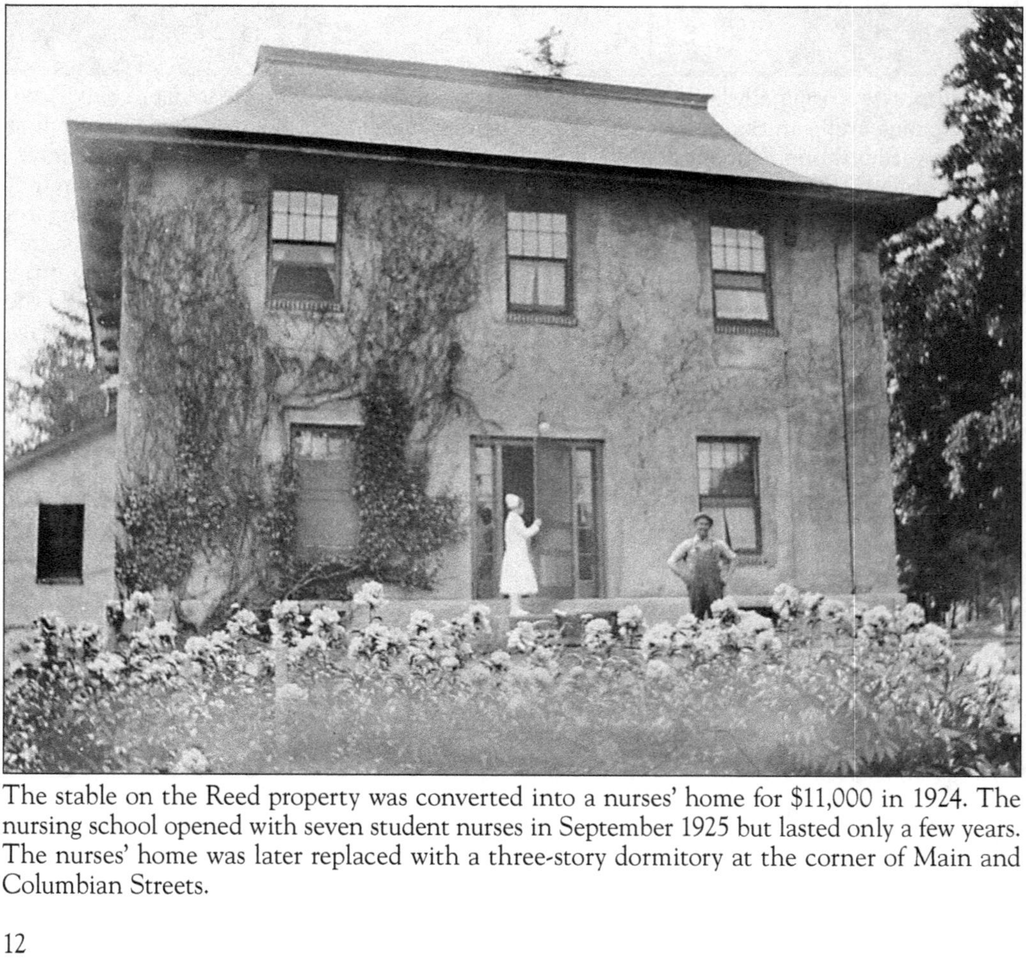

The stable on the Reed property was converted into a nurses' home for $11,000 in 1924. The nursing school opened with seven student nurses in September 1925 but lasted only a few years. The nurses' home was later replaced with a three-story dormitory at the corner of Main and Columbian Streets.

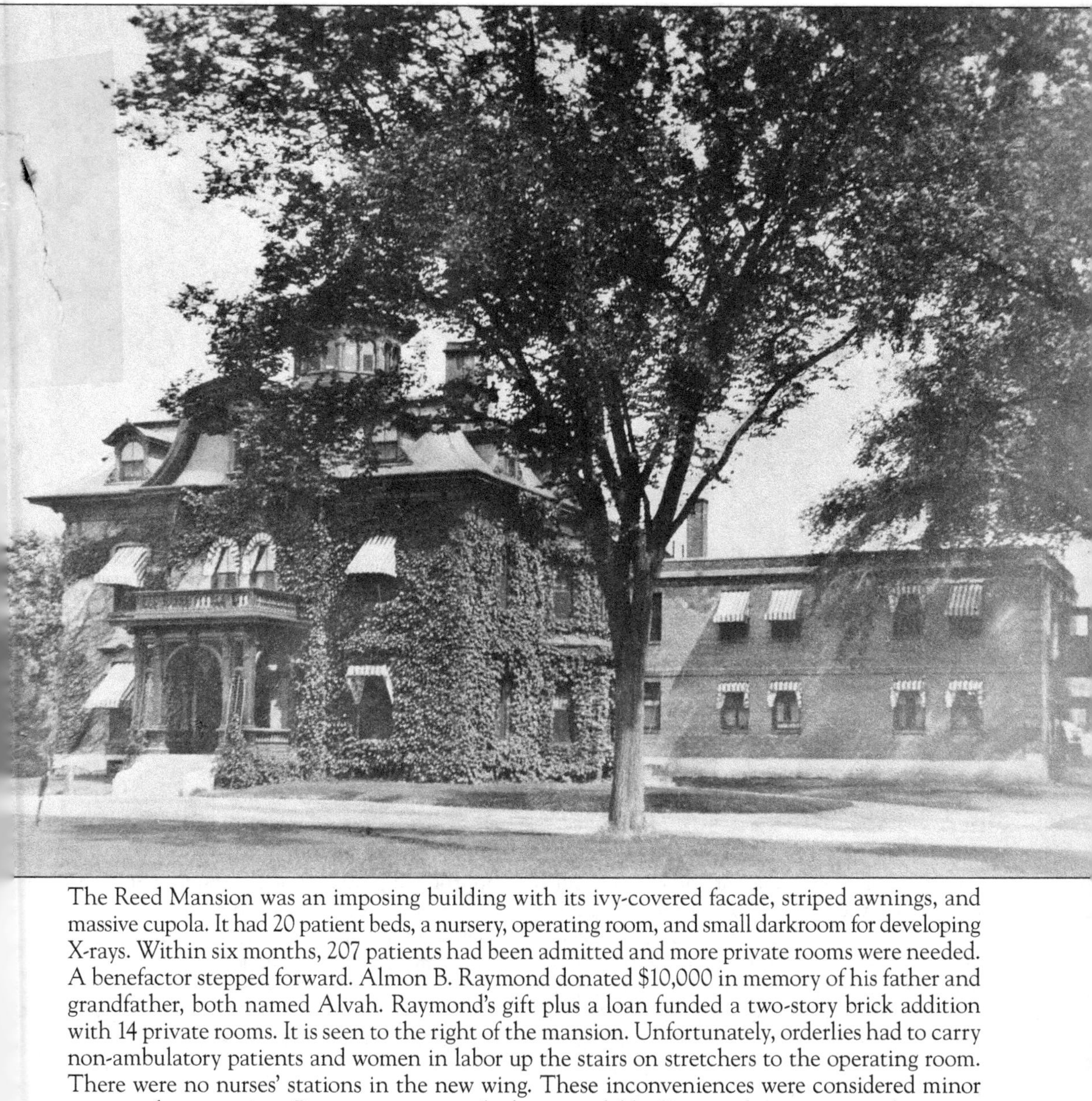

The Reed Mansion was an imposing building with its ivy-covered facade, striped awnings, and massive cupola. It had 20 patient beds, a nursery, operating room, and small darkroom for developing X-rays. Within six months, 207 patients had been admitted and more private rooms were needed. A benefactor stepped forward. Almon B. Raymond donated $10,000 in memory of his father and grandfather, both named Alvah. Raymond's gift plus a loan funded a two-story brick addition with 14 private rooms. It is seen to the right of the mansion. Unfortunately, orderlies had to carry non-ambulatory patients and women in labor up the stairs on stretchers to the operating room. There were no nurses' stations in the new wing. These inconveniences were considered minor compared to a trip into Boston, assuming a bed was available. Despite these accommodations to what had long been a residence, Weymouth Hospital thrived.

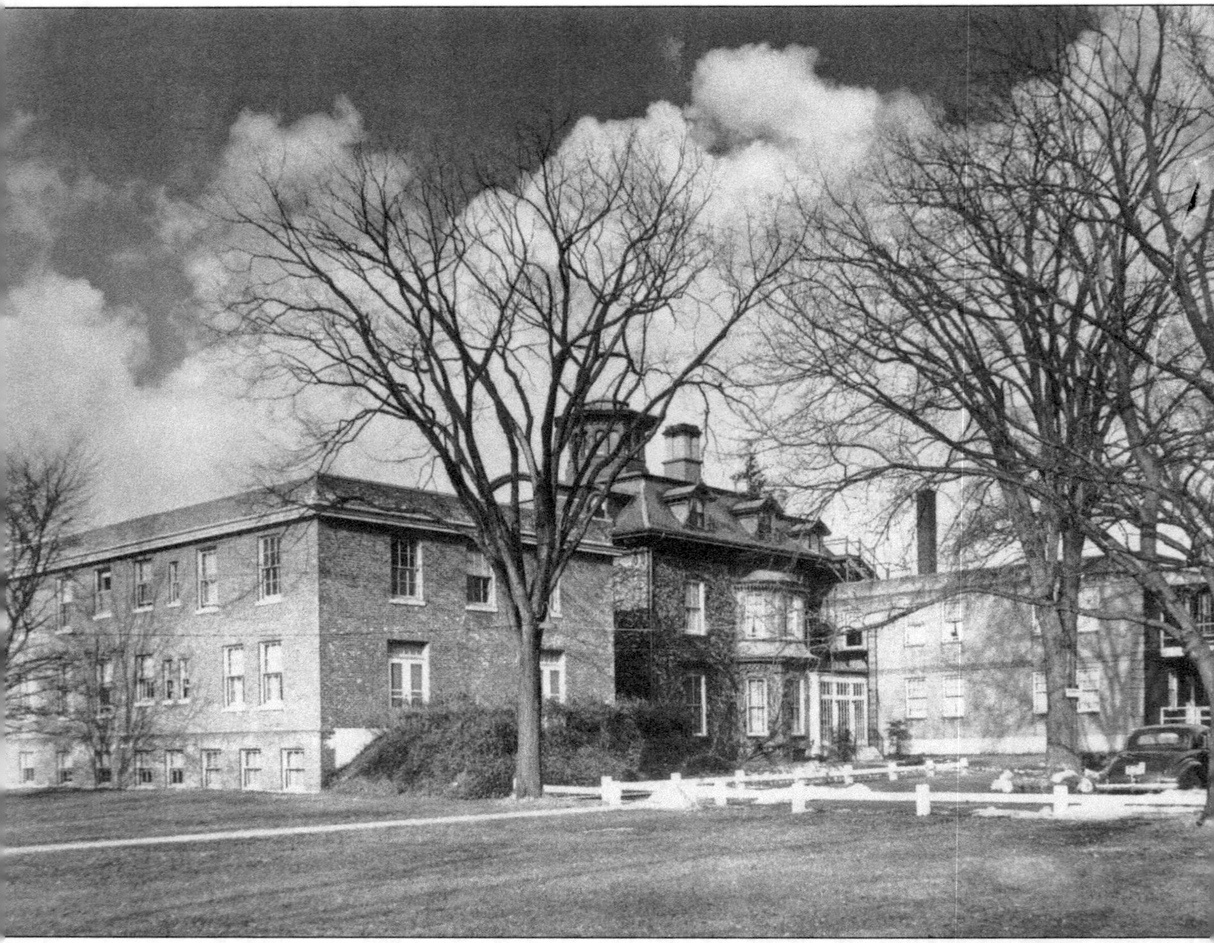

This photograph shows the Public Works Administration (PWA) building left of the Reed Mansion (and the Raymond Wing at the right). Built in 1936, the wing was funded through a $60,000 PWA loan, the first to a private organization. Much-needed surgery suites and maternity wards were added to relieve overcrowding. An accident room and ambulance entrance were located more efficiently on the ground floor. Installing an elevator meant that staff no longer had to carry patients unable to walk up and down stairs on stretchers. When the PWA building opened in 1936, bed capacity leaped to 90, almost three times larger than in 1923. In 1941, Weymouth Wool Scouring Company president Bryan Leonard donated $10,000 to renovate the overcrowded nursery unit in memory of his parents. Although no longer visible from the street, the Administration Building continues to be used for offices.

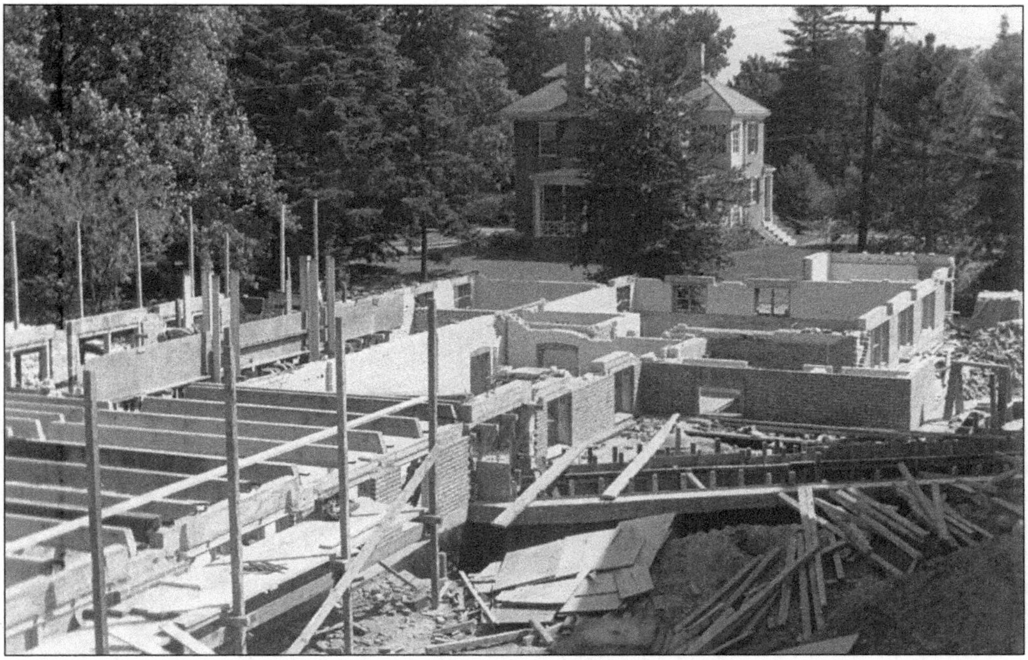

The federal government initially approved a grant-loan from the Federal Works Agency in 1941. A request to purchase the materials was denied after the Federal Civil Defense Authority refused to recognize Weymouth as a strategic area, despite the naval air station and nearby suppliers of war materials. After years of negotiating, the government awarded $247,750 to construct a separate 36-bed, two-story building with facilities for maternity and pediatrics. With structural steel and reinforced concrete scarce, it was built using mill construction and wooden framing. The trustees wanted to change the hospital's name to reflect the larger service area from which they hoped to draw financial support. In 1945, the name South Shore Hospital was accepted and appeared for the first time on the Center Building.

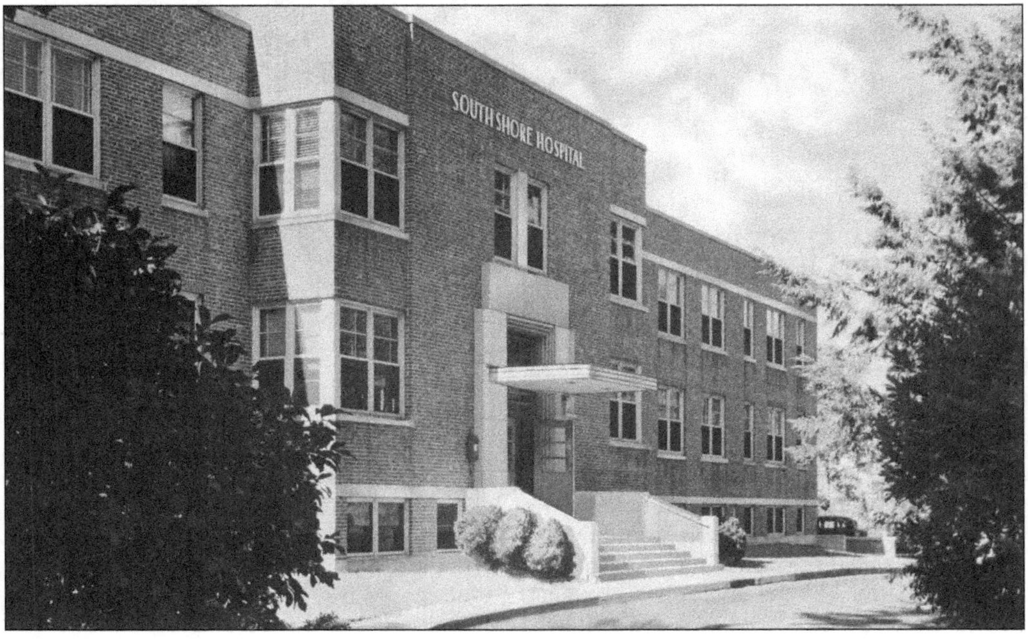

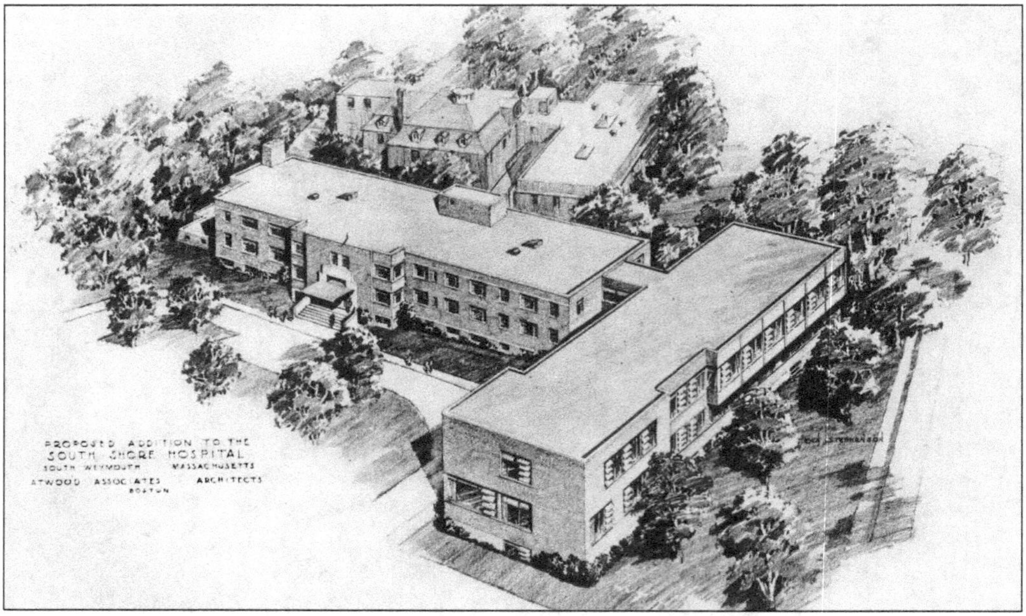
PROPOSED ADDITION TO THE
SOUTH SHORE HOSPITAL
SOUTH WEYMOUTH MASSACHUSETTS
ATWOOD ASSOCIATES ARCHITECTS
BOSTON

At an angle to the Center Building, the West Wing contained 152 maternity beds, later 188 beds, including 57 bassinets. The hospital continued to feel pressure for more beds. Within days of opening, 300 patients were waiting for beds. Within a year, 1,903 babies were born in the wing. The new emergency room, the first in the region open 24 hours a day, treated 6,350 patients the first year.

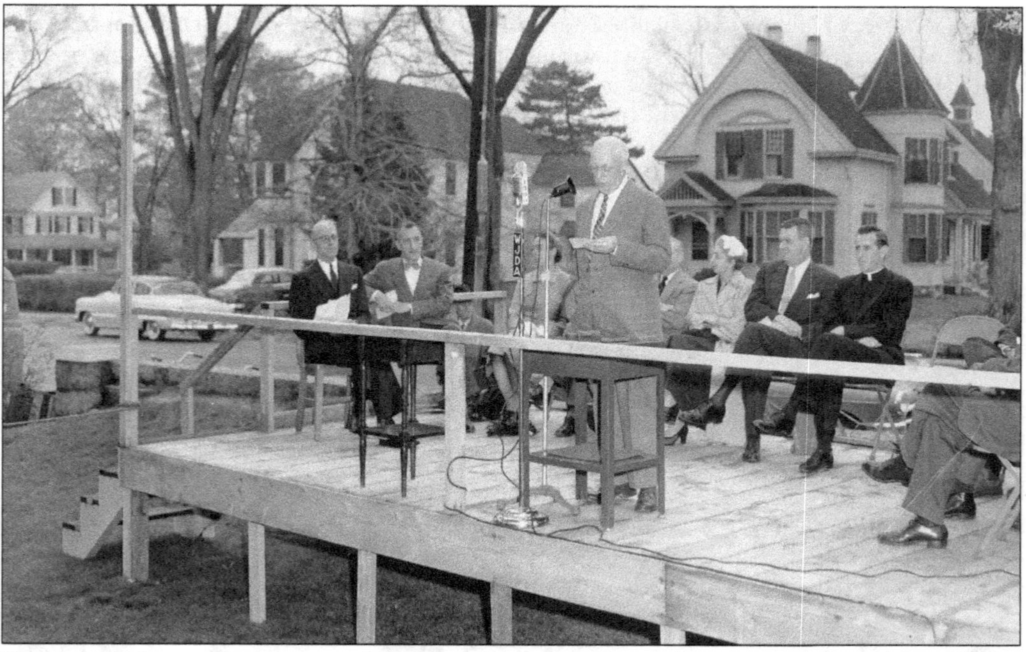

Expansion of maternity care owed much to Dr. Robert Ryan, shown seated second from left at the West Wing dedication. Both he and the hospital earned national recognition for expert care when he delivered the Manning quadruplets. His reputation opened doors in Washington, and he obtained crucial financing. A 37-bed pediatric unit opened in 1957, and the treatment room was dedicated in memory of World War II Pacific casualty Walton Killam Rodgers.

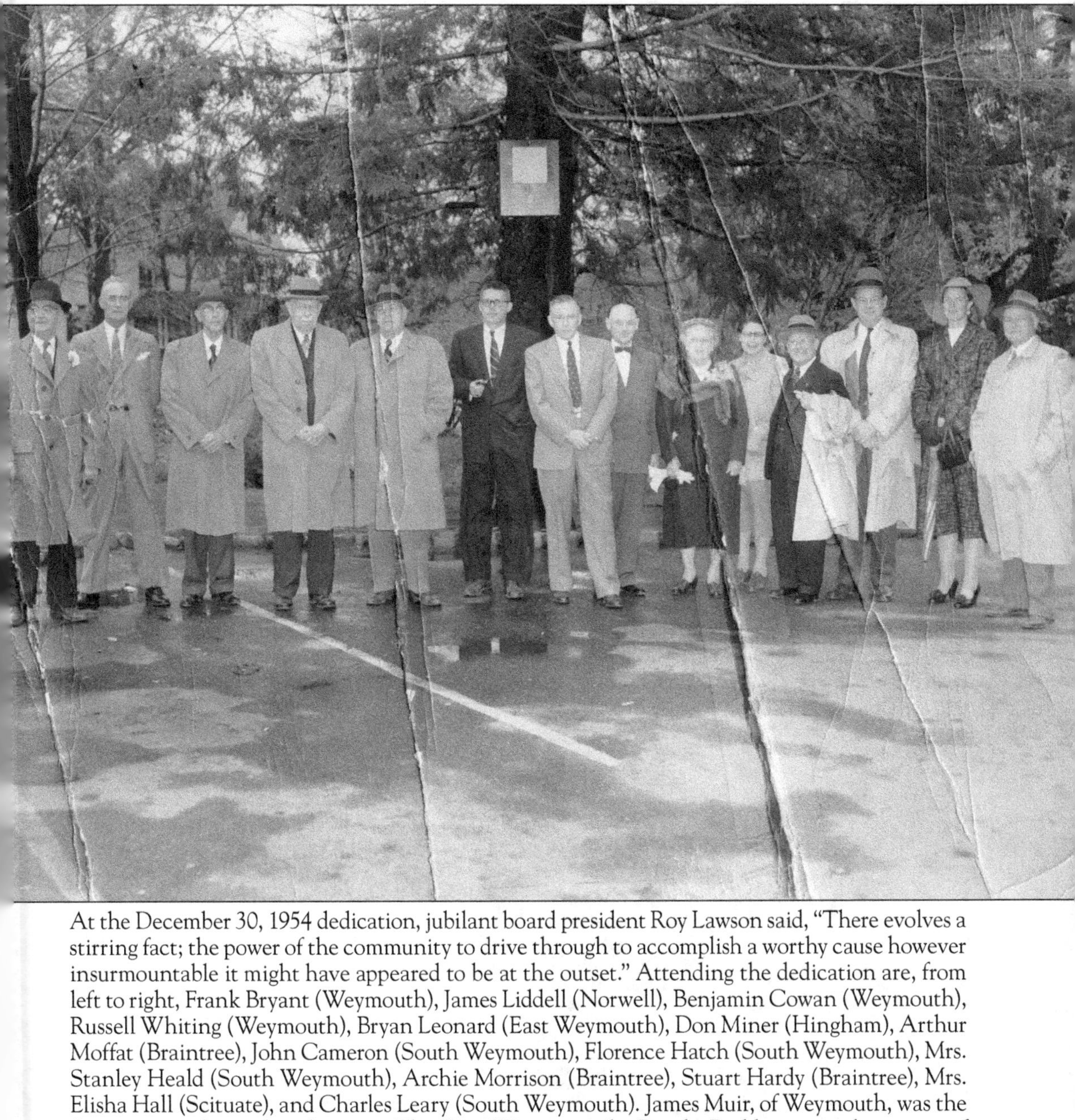

At the December 30, 1954 dedication, jubilant board president Roy Lawson said, "There evolves a stirring fact; the power of the community to drive through to accomplish a worthy cause however insurmountable it might have appeared to be at the outset." Attending the dedication are, from left to right, Frank Bryant (Weymouth), James Liddell (Norwell), Benjamin Cowan (Weymouth), Russell Whiting (Weymouth), Bryan Leonard (East Weymouth), Don Miner (Hingham), Arthur Moffat (Braintree), John Cameron (South Weymouth), Florence Hatch (South Weymouth), Mrs. Stanley Heald (South Weymouth), Archie Morrison (Braintree), Stuart Hardy (Braintree), Mrs. Elisha Hall (Scituate), and Charles Leary (South Weymouth). James Muir, of Weymouth, was the first patient admitted to the wing. The West Wing, now the Brooks Building, is at the corner of Main and Columbian Streets and is one of the most visible buildings on the campus. It houses physical and cardiac rehabilitation, the pharmacy, and administrative offices.

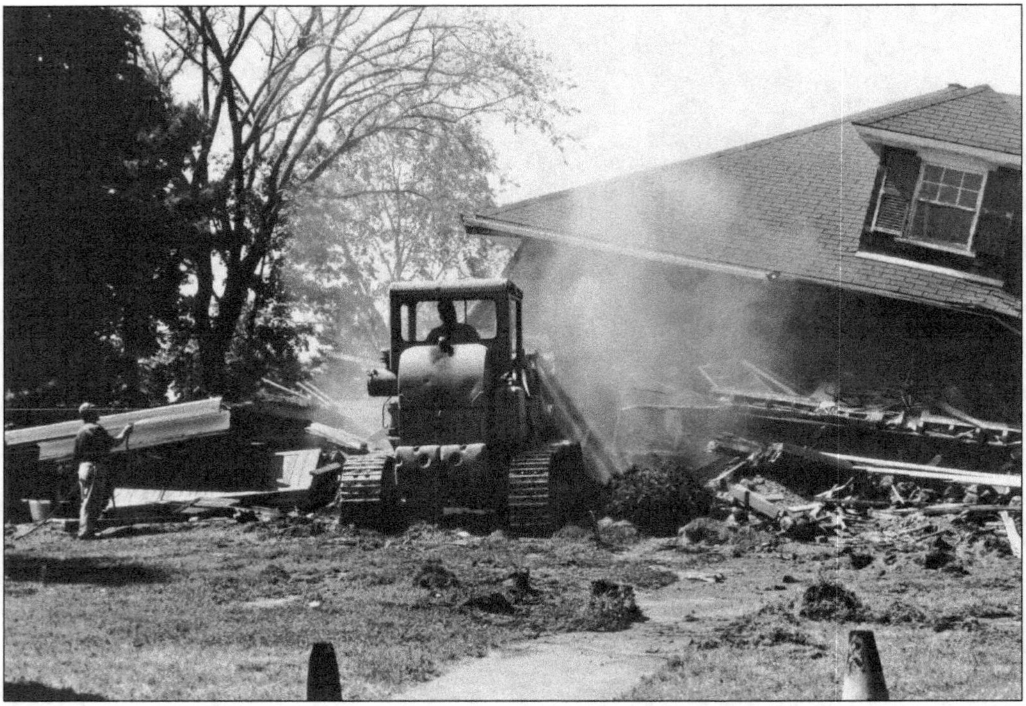

The hospital bought the former homes of Dr. George Emerson and Stetson Shoe president Charles Heald. The property included a small apple orchard on Fogg Road. The buildings were bulldozed to make way for the Laban Pratt Building and much-needed parking. The hospital continued its pattern of a major addition nearly every decade.

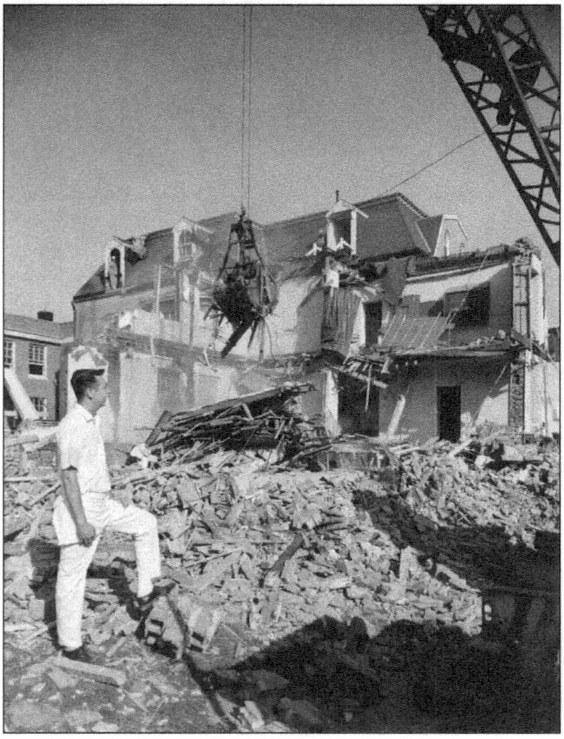

The pre–Civil War Reed Mansion had been a residence, chapel, and hospital. When demolished in 1967, it was well over 100 years old and impractical for hospital use. Assistant Food Service Director William Molisse, of Weymouth, watched the demolition of the Raymond Wing. The mansard roof of the mansion is about to be leveled to make way for the new Laban Pratt Building.

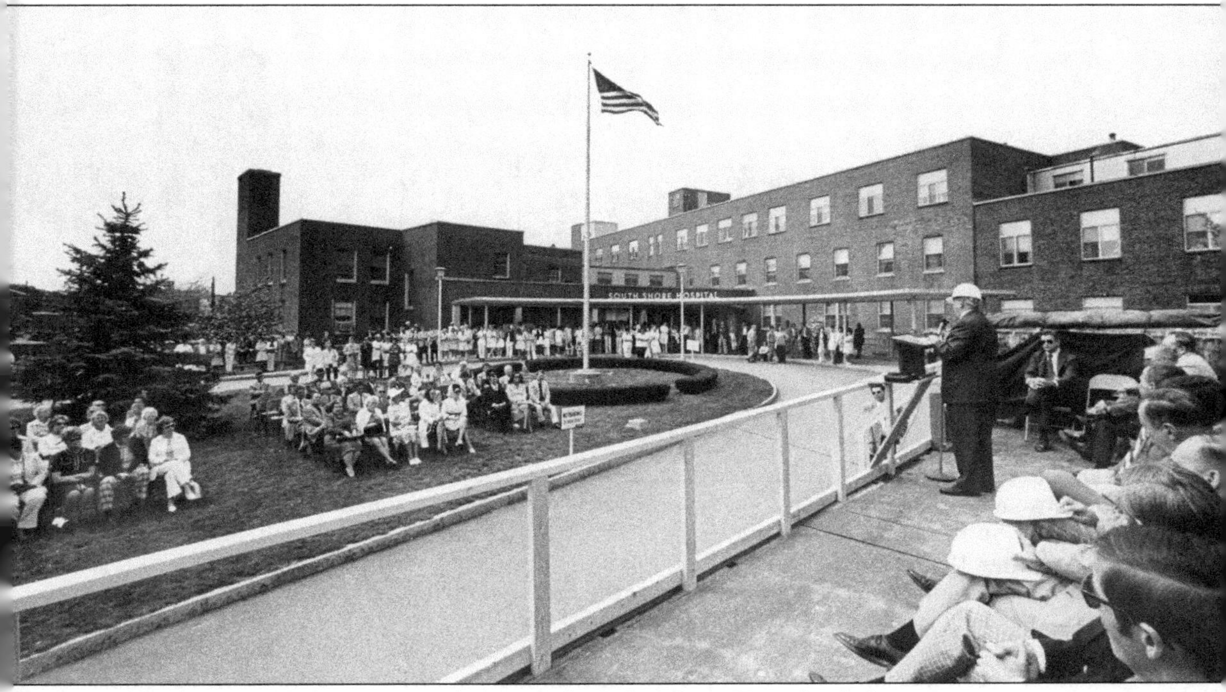

Local leaders prevailed in court to designate the Laban Pratt Trust funds for a new wing at the hospital instead of a separate facility in Weymouth. The building was also funded through federal Hill-Burton grants and public donations. A trustee noted, "It was a long, cold winter, but the work went on. Portable heaters and acres of plastic kept sand and cement at workable temperatures, and were of some help in enabling the construction workers to keep going." This three-story addition was part of a four-phase, $4.4 million construction. A fourth floor was added to the Center Building, the laboratory and pharmacy expanded, and a new cardiac unit opened. In 1969, trustees voted to add three new floors to the Pratt Building with the top floor reserved for one of the region's first intensive care units. When the building opened, daily rates were $59 (private room), $50 (two-bed, semiprivate room), and $45 (four-bed, semiprivate room). Pratt North's rates were slightly higher. Intensive care beds were $75 a day. The hospital had 245 beds at this time. This photograph shows the 1967 dedication.

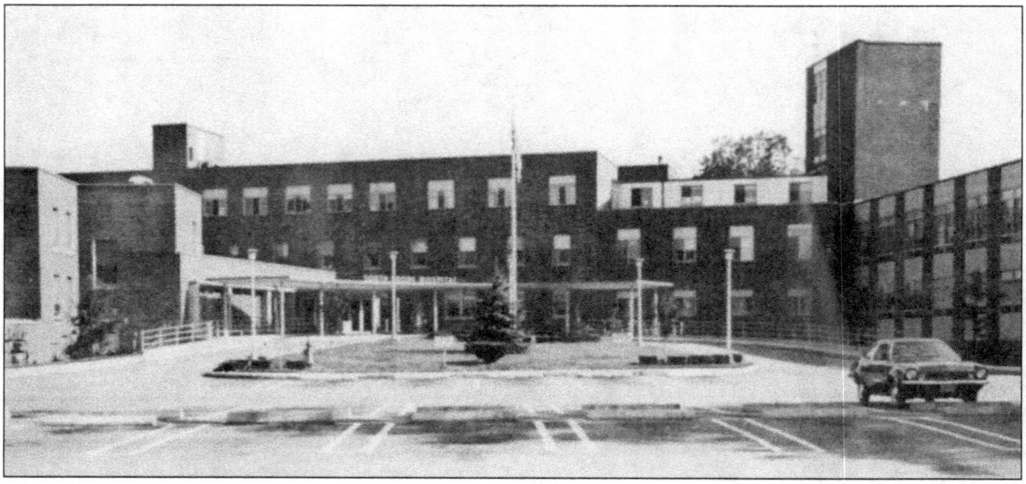

The above view was familiar to patients arriving at the hospital's main entrance on Fogg Road in 1972. In the aerial photograph below, Main Street (Route 18) is on the left, and Columbian Street is at the top of the campus. Surrounding the sweeping driveway are, from left to right, the power plant, the 1955 West Wing (now the Brooks Building) at an angle and connected to both the 1936 Administration Building and the 1945 Center Building. The new Pratt Building is at the right of the campus. In 1969, three floors were added to the Pratt Building. The hospital had 340 beds, including 32 in the intensive care/coronary unit. This unit was staffed 24 hours a day by board-certified physicians specially trained in intensive care medicine. A year later, the Level II special care nursery opened. There were 2,500 births, and the emergency room cared for 60,000 patients.

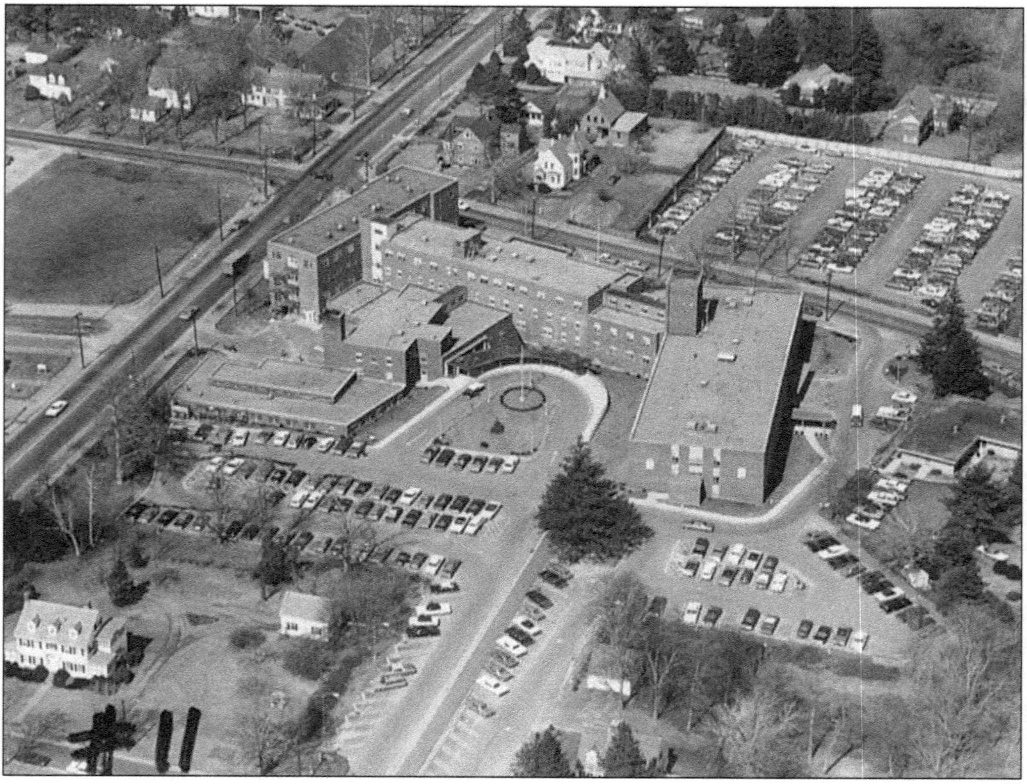

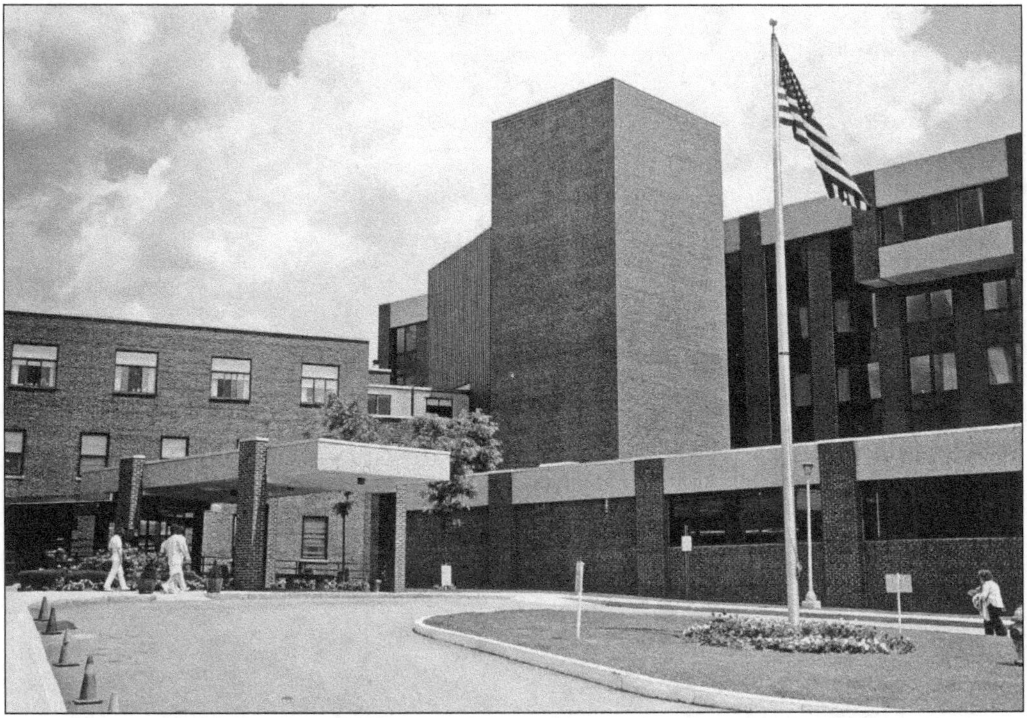

The hospital continued to need more patient rooms, outpatient clinics, and administrative space. This 1976 photograph (above) shows a redesigned and more imposing front entrance on Fogg Road. Construction started on the Chassis Building, which was partially wrapped around the Laban Pratt Building, as seen below in the aerial photograph. Later, the Emerson Building (patient rooms, dining room, and a new main entrance) was built over the Administration Building. The Emilson Center (emergency, maternity, and surgery) was constructed over and next to the Chassis Building. In this aerial photograph looking north, the Administration Building and main entrance is bracketed by the West Wing and Center Building.

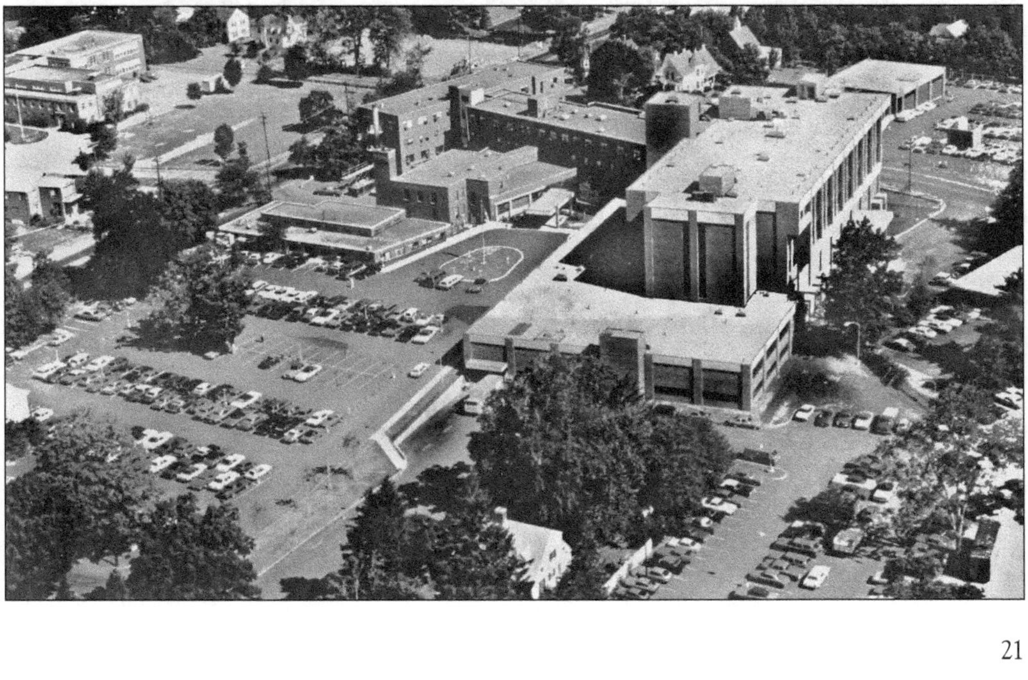

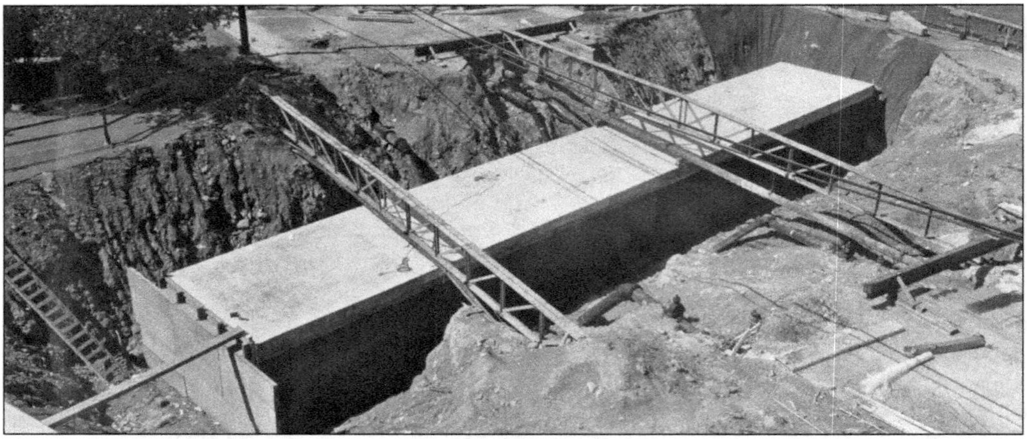

In 1976, engineers designed a tunnel under Columbian Street to connect the campus to the new power plant. Traffic was diverted for many months onto what is now a hospital parking lot. This view looking north was taken from the Laban Pratt Building. A second, larger tunnel was added from the W. Torrey and Doris Little Center 17 years later.

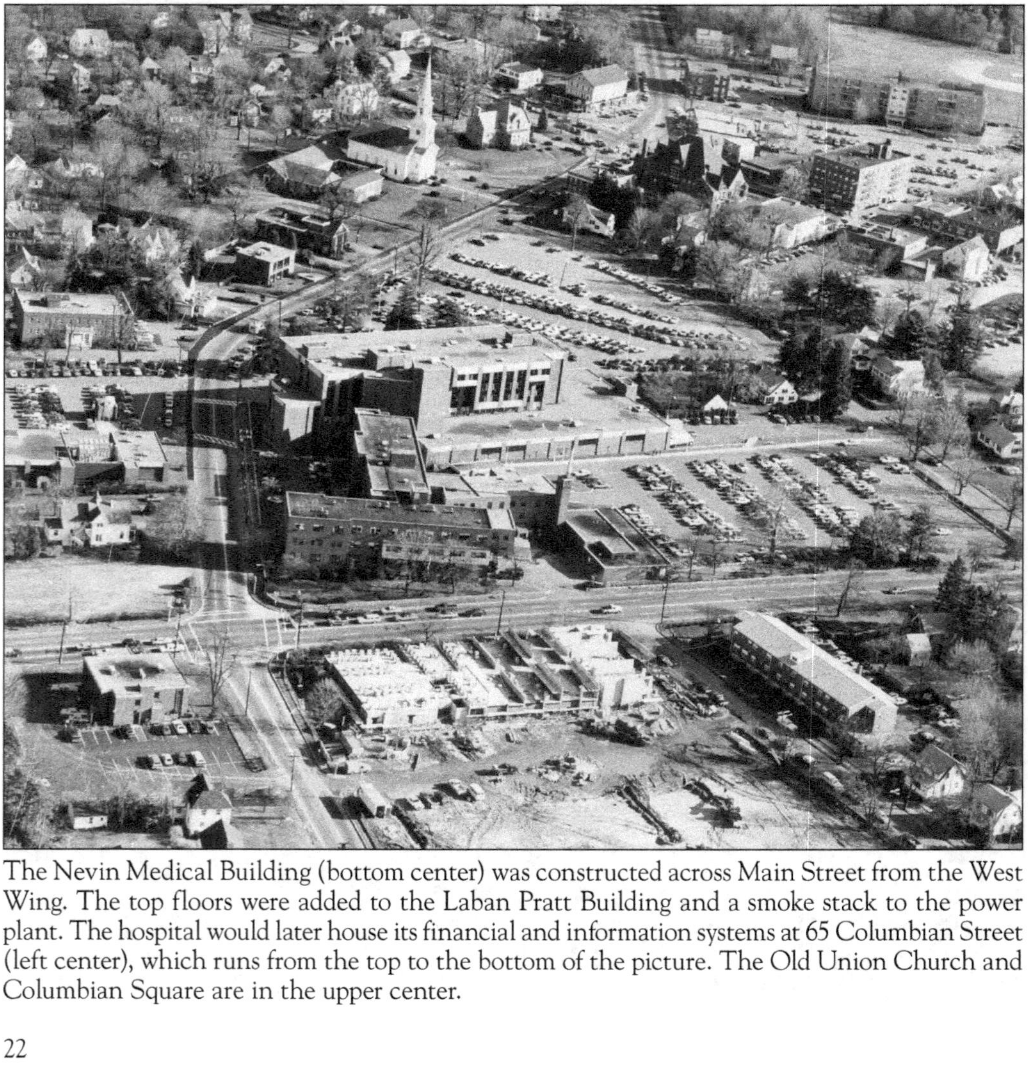

The Nevin Medical Building (bottom center) was constructed across Main Street from the West Wing. The top floors were added to the Laban Pratt Building and a smoke stack to the power plant. The hospital would later house its financial and information systems at 65 Columbian Street (left center), which runs from the top to the bottom of the picture. The Old Union Church and Columbian Square are in the upper center.

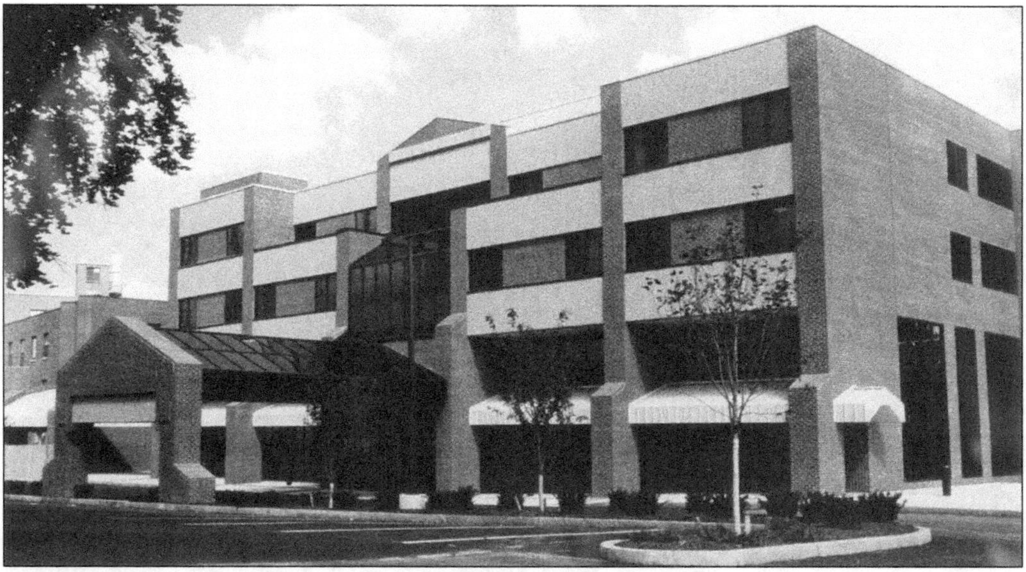

In 1989, the Emerson Building was named after Dr. George Emerson, a hospital founder who had died a few years previously. Facing Main Street, it became the hub of the hospital and was the main entrance for 22 years. The Emerson Building contained two floors of patient rooms, the main dining room, and support space. The hospital entered an era of unprecedented growth. A year after the Emerson Building opened, plans were announced for a new building that increased accommodations 20 percent, up from 2,200 a year, and included a much-needed new emergency department. Although the campus appears to be fully built out, through creative design, the hospital added the Emilson (1991), Little (1993), Emilson expansion (2003), and F.X. Messina (2003) Buildings. In 2011, the 60 patient beds in Emerson were doubled with an addition to the existing building and the inclusion of two new floors.

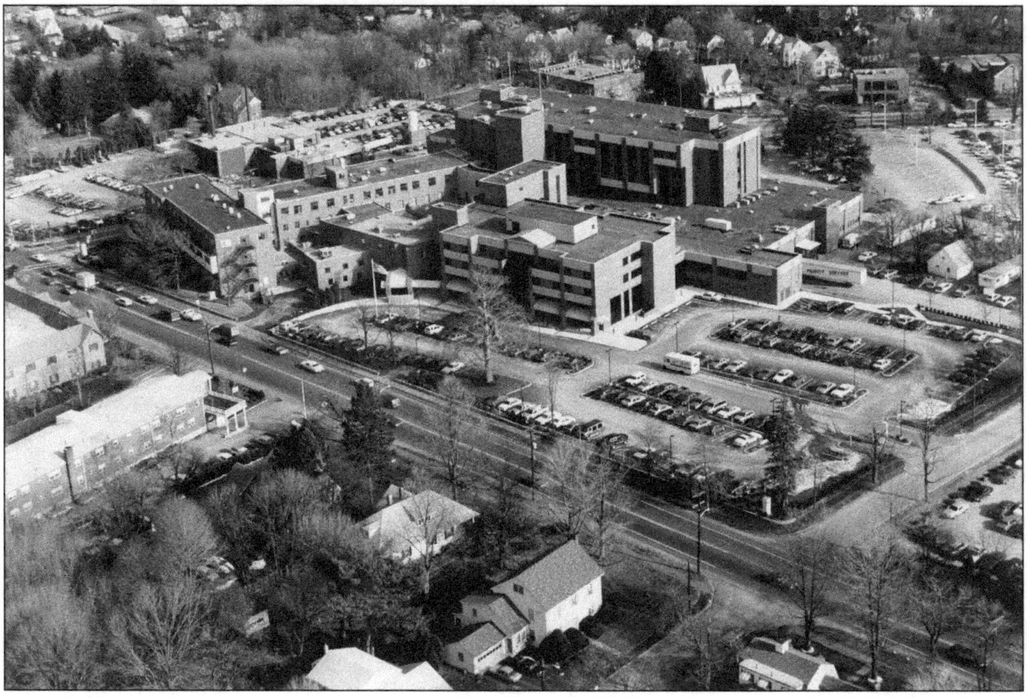

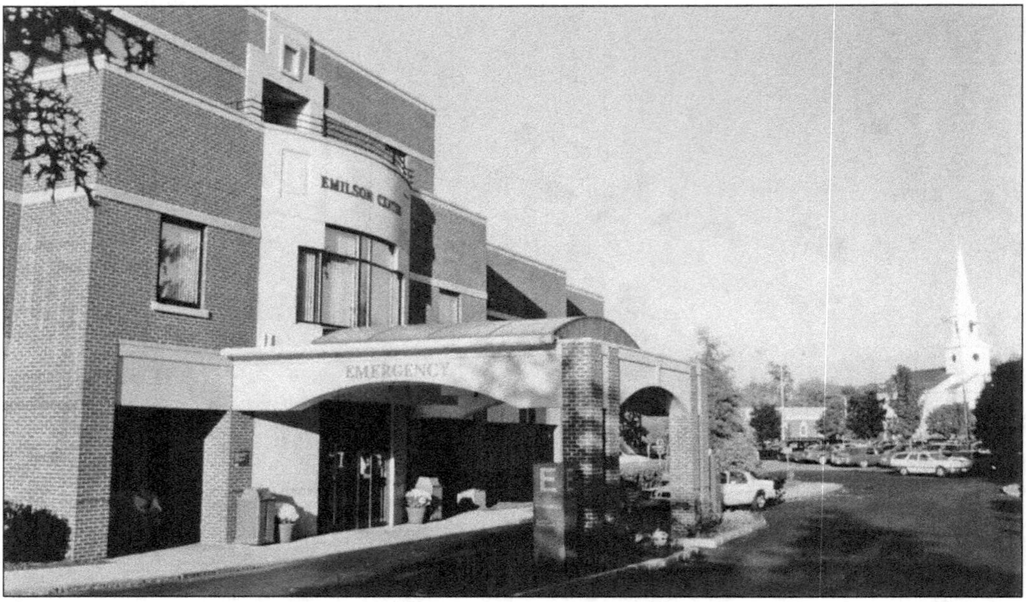

Honoring C. Herbert and Paulie Emilson, this building housed the region's largest maternity service, which was capable of handling 4,500 births a year. Its emergency department handled 60,000 visits annually, an improvement over the 1967 building (15,000 visits). Within a few years, it proved too small, and an 81-bed unit opened in the new F.X. Messina Center (85,000 visits). The Emilson expansion and Messina construction cost $65 million, then the hospital's largest capital project.

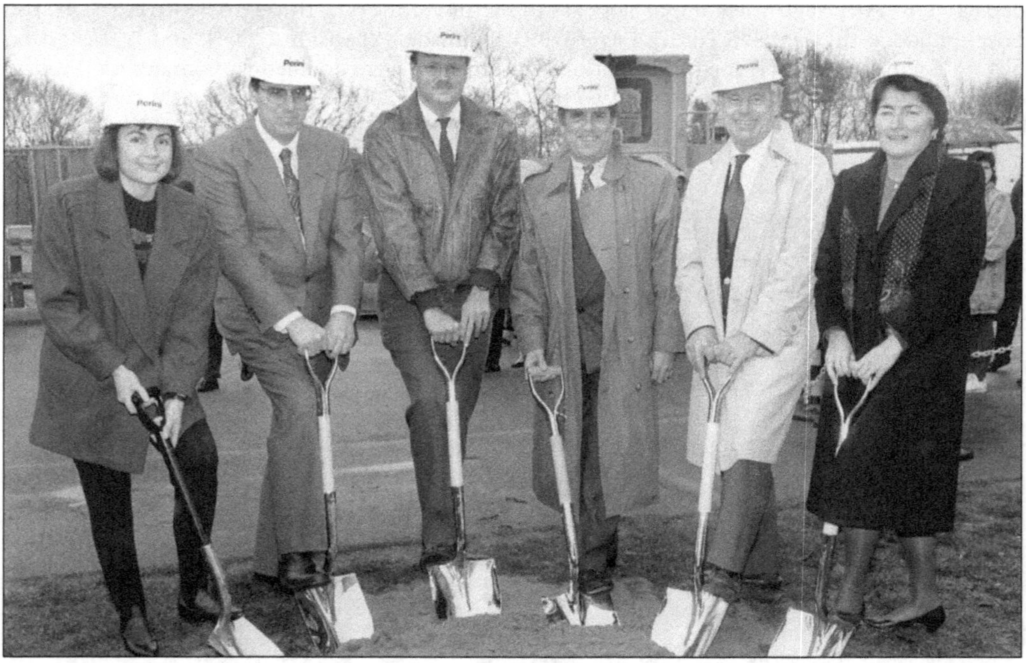

Laboratory employees joined officials at a groundbreaking to kick off the laboratory modernization and expansion in a building later to be named the W. Torrey and Doris Little Center. From left to right are Debbie Zeller (medical technician), Dr. Dante Cannarozzi (chairman of pathology), Eric Potter (supervisor of hematology), David Hannan (president and chief executive officer), James Bristol Jr. (board chairman), and Rosemary Stefani (assistant director of Laboratory Services).

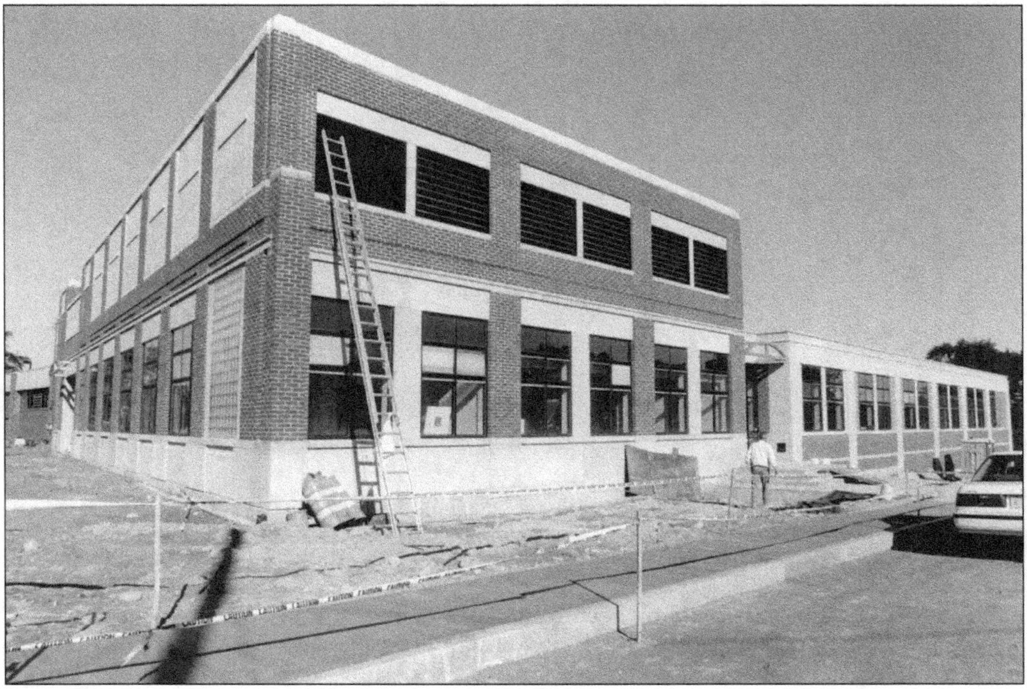

The Little Center houses an expanded laboratory in which hundreds of thousands of samples are examined annually. They are transported from operating suites via pneumatic tubes within seconds. Opened in the Fall of 1993, the 33,000-square-foot, two-story building also contains materials management, with millions of medical supplies and equipment passing through it each year.

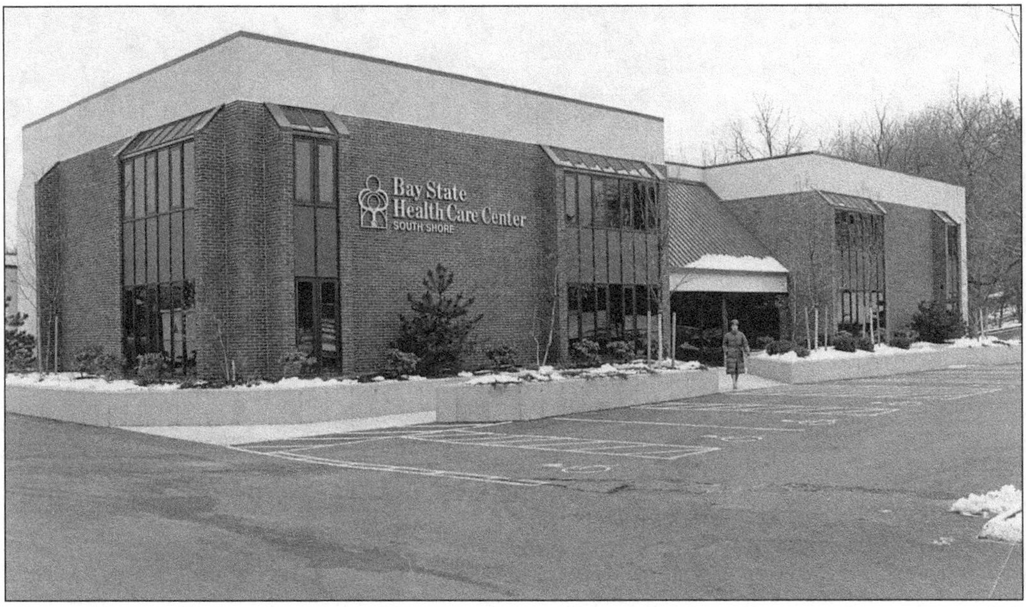

The building at 780 Main Street in Weymouth was a Purity Supreme Supermarket, a dance club and function hall, and an outpatient surgery center for Bay State Healthcare, pictured in 1986. South Shore Hospital obtained the master lease and later purchased the building. It became an outpatient surgical center and physician offices before outpatient orthopedic surgery was moved to the Center for Orthopedics, Spine, and Sports Medicine in Hingham.

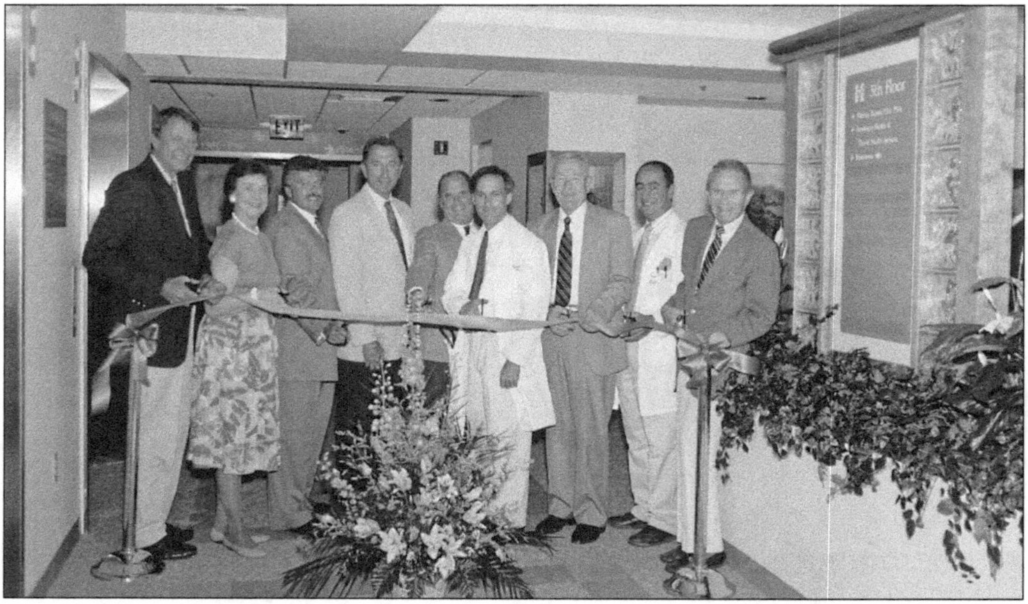

The five-story Laban Pratt Building housed the largest cardiology and radiology departments and the first Level II neonatal care unit in southeastern Massachusetts. At a 1994 ribbon-cutting are, from left to right, Director David Chase, Friends of South Shore Hospital president Barbara MacSwan, Director Richard Nash, board chairman Arthur Sharp, hospital president and Chief Executive Officer David Hannan, Director of Cardiology Dr. Anthony Marks, Director David Jones, Dr. James Bezreh, and Director Henry Hoffman.

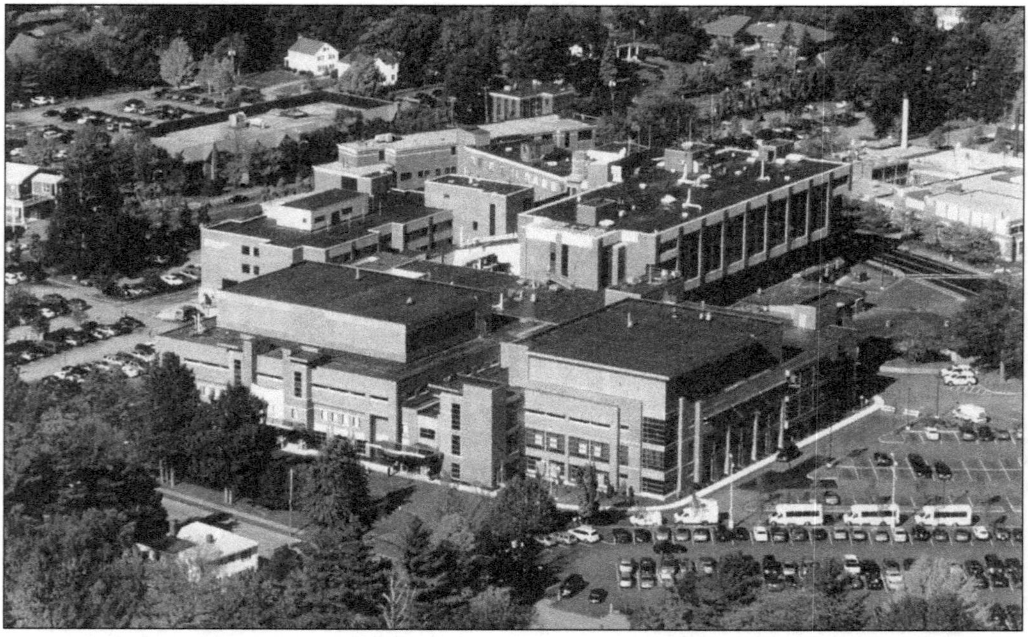

Pictured in 2002, the Weymouth campus would later include a $90 million cancer center, garage, and a two-story, 60-bed addition and bump-out to the Emerson Building. With little space available on campus, the hospital opened a new Center for Orthopedics, Spine, and Sports Medicine in Hingham in 2011. Off-campus facilities include outpatient services for women and children in Weymouth and a mammography center in Cohasset.

Two

Medical Staff

"With Undiminished Energy"

W. Carleton Barnes so described the medical staff in a 1933 annual report. The hospital's first medical staff included Drs. George Emerson, Frederick Doucette, Wallace Drake, and Cornelius Sullivan. Initially, only Weymouth physicians were included. Soon afterward, the staff organized themselves as active members and those with courtesy privileges. Bylaws revised privileges in 1929 following a recommendation by the American Medical Association that required physicians to meet specific criteria. In 1933, Weymouth Hospital was fully approved by the American College of Surgeons—a notable achievement for the nine-year-old hospital. Over the years, in-house specialists replaced consultants for specialized surgery, orthopedics, and maternity care. From the original four physicians, the staff grew to include physicians from world-renowned medical schools and academic medical centers who earned privileges to practice at the hospital.

Medical staff presidents were George Emerson, Frederick Doucette, Wallace Drake, Cornelius Sullivan, Clifford Danforth, Daniel Bailey, John Peckham, Robert Ross, Harris Bowmar, Harold Ripley, Arsham Alemian, Robert Ryan, Raymond Vinal, Edward Howley, Burton Elder, John Hopkins, Folke Wiklund, Kenneth Dalton, George F. Emerson, Arthur Sullivan, Edward Connolly, Archie Keigan, and Philip Landry.

Additional presidents were Edward Nalband, Donald Tardiff, Wallace Kemp, James Dolphin, John Peters, Grant Dixey, Paul Duggan, John McConville, Robert Seidel, John O'Brien, Charles Rounds, Albert Marcus, Arthur Garceau, Richard Alemian, Bartley Cilento, Kenneth Travis; James Penza, Stephen O'Connor, David Rudolph, James Everett, Charles Gaughan, Timothy McGinn, Frederick Ayer, Robert Brancale, Russell Kelley, Edward Nalband, Giovanni Ferrante, Brian Battista, and Clifford Breslow.

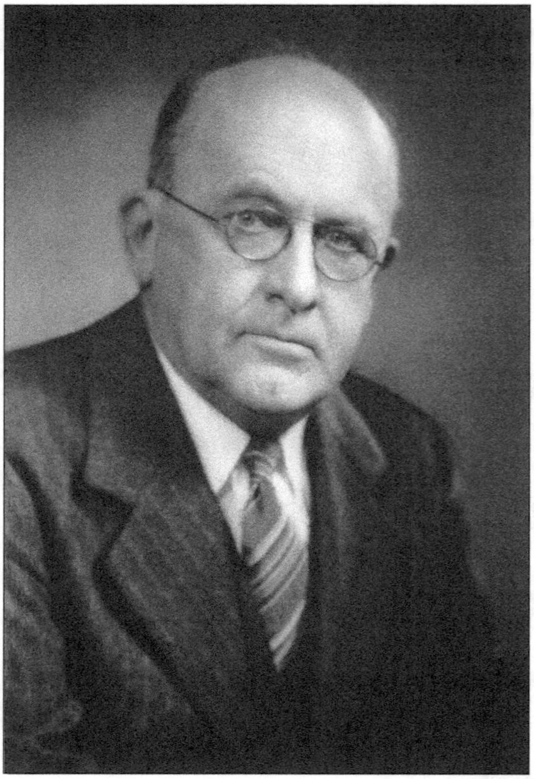

Dr. George E. Emerson and three other Weymouth physicians formed the hospital's first medical staff in 1922. Emerson collected fees from patients and distributed proceeds daily to specialists. He was also board treasurer. Emerson died December 26, 1962, at age 82. With his son and grandson, also medical staff members over the years, an Emerson has always been involved in the hospital.

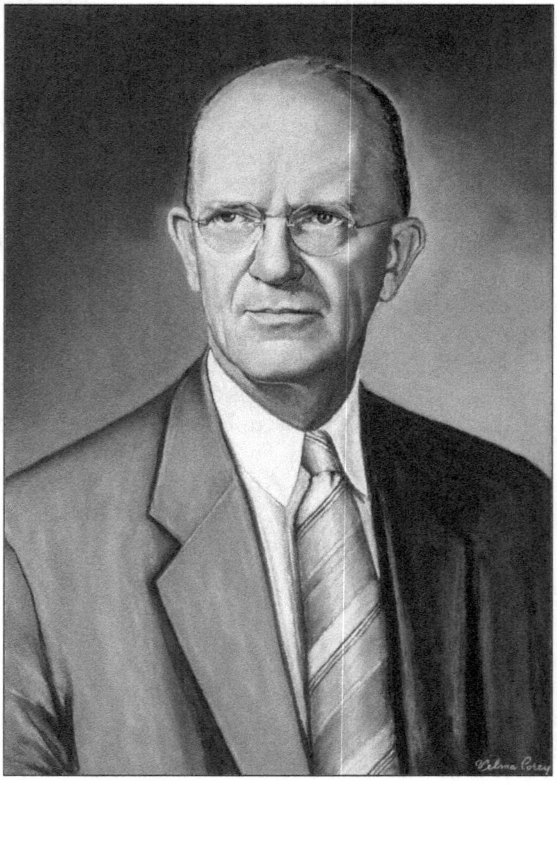

Of the four original staff physicians, Dr. Wallace Drake was the last to retire from the medical staff. A North Weymouth resident, Drake graduated from Harvard Medical School in 1918. His career spanned enormous growth in programs, technology, and the expansion of the campus. He was an elder statesman to the medical staff. He died in 1971. This portrait by Velma Corey is displayed in the hospital's medical staff lounge.

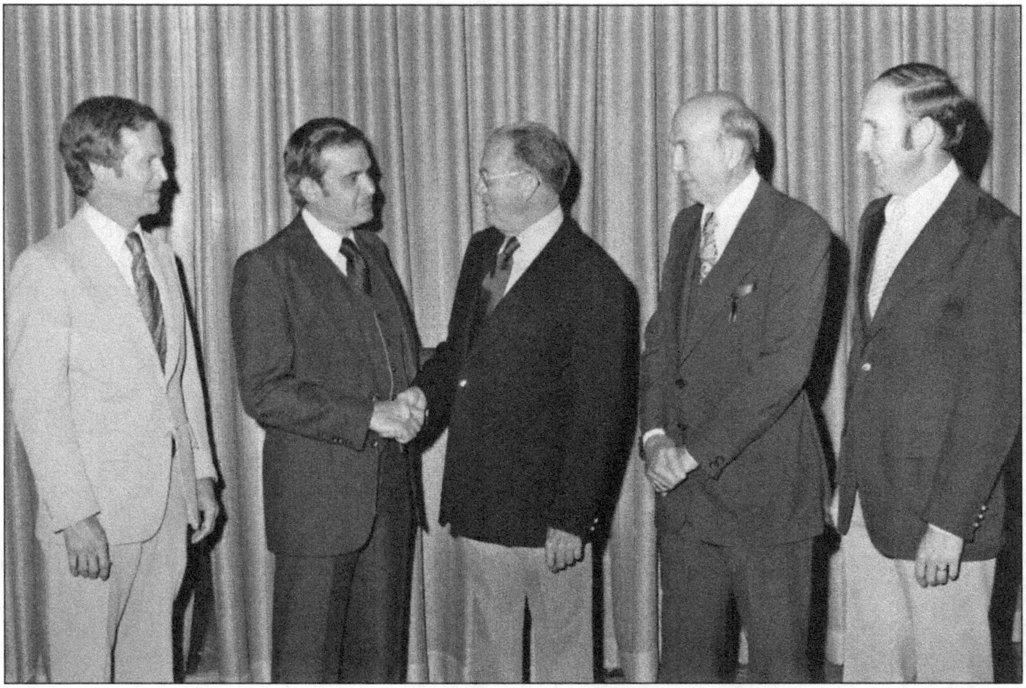

Founder George Emerson was honored at the hospital's 50th anniversary. From left to right, medical staff presidents Drs. Paul Duggan and Philip Landry welcome Emerson sons and grandson Drs. George, Ralph, and Geoffrey. A $34 million addition was named for Emerson 15 years later. With 60 beds, it was three times larger than the original Weymouth Hospital. In 2011, construction started to add another 60 beds to the building.

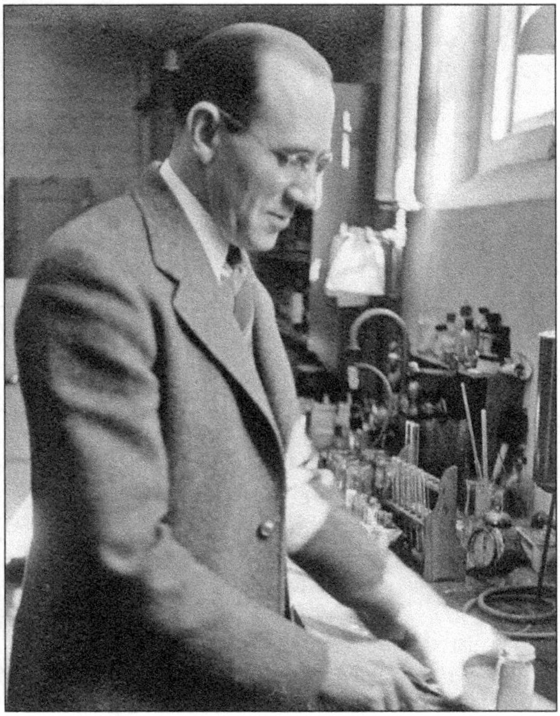

Dr. James Cameron works in the laboratory in a three-piece suit in 1939. He was admitted to the hospital's staff when it expanded from the original four to ten physicians. At the time, the hospital's 94 beds were at 90 percent occupancy, a rate that burdened the small laboratory. Dr. Cameron likely performed his own tests.

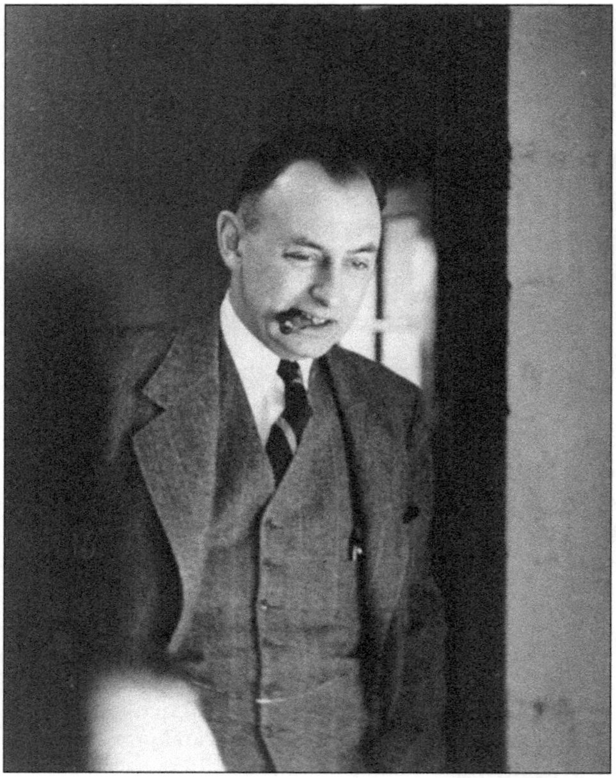

Dr. John Peckham, of North Abington, appears just before enlisting during World War II. He returned to serve as medical staff president, the first to regularly represent the medical staff at hospital board meetings. The hospital was booming with 4,000 patients. Peckham helped improve procedures for medical records and established an autopsy room.

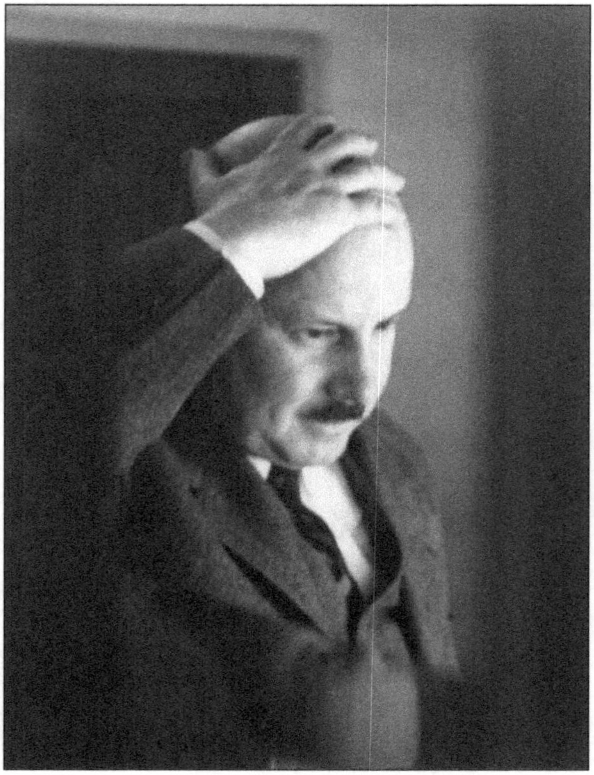

In this 1941 photograph, Dr. Herbert Hulse appears in typical attire of physicians: a heavy, three-piece wool suit and regimental tie, all designed to inspire confidence. Later that year, he would wear a naval uniform as one of 18 physicians who enlisted. The war caused shortages of physicians and nurses while demand for care exploded.

Dr. Raymond Vinal, of Norwell, was medical staff president from 1957 to 1958. After two Norwell youngsters died from polio, the opening of school was delayed until Vinal could obtain the Salk vaccine and start inoculations. During the summers, South Shore Hospital lent nurses to assist Boston hospitals overwhelmed with polio patients.

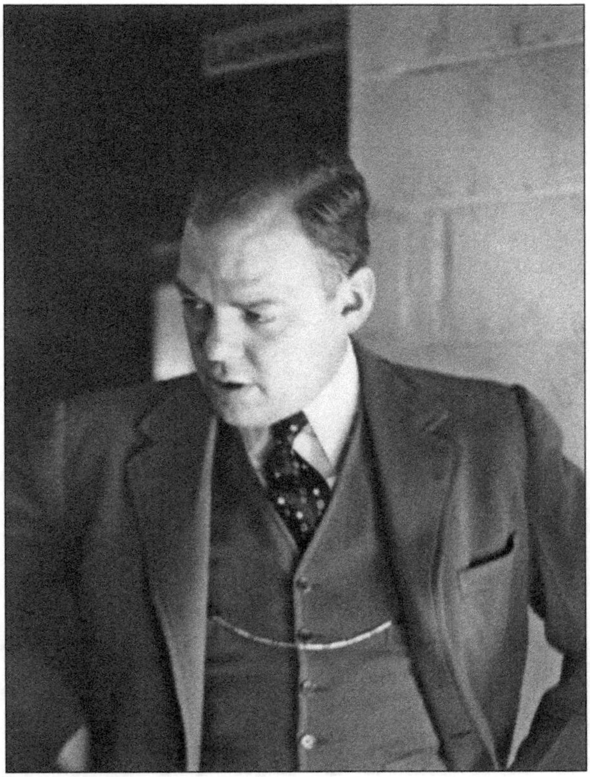

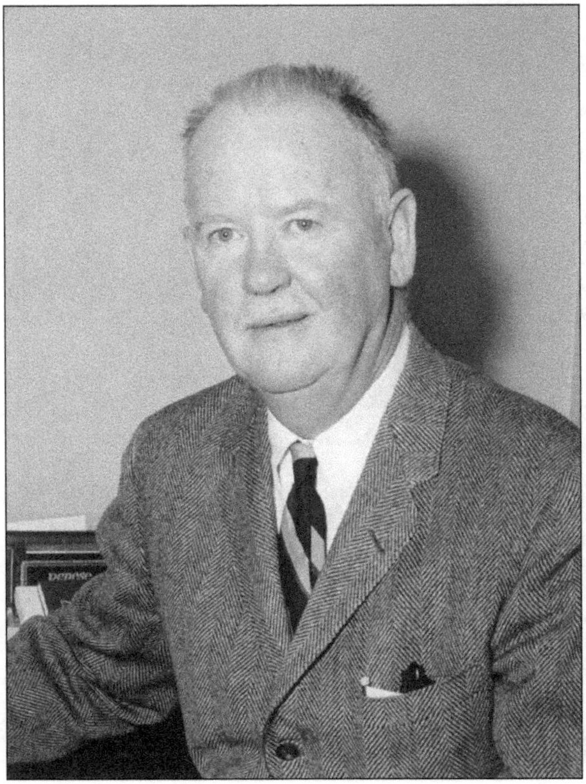

Dr. Kenneth Dalton was medical staff president in 1966. He oversaw a prepackaged emergency hospital, a Cold War staple that was revived during the Cuban Missile Crisis. This hospital-in-a-container quickly converted into a minimal but completely functional 200-bed hospital, with wards, operating suites, and laboratory that could replace a damaged or destroyed hospital "post-attack."

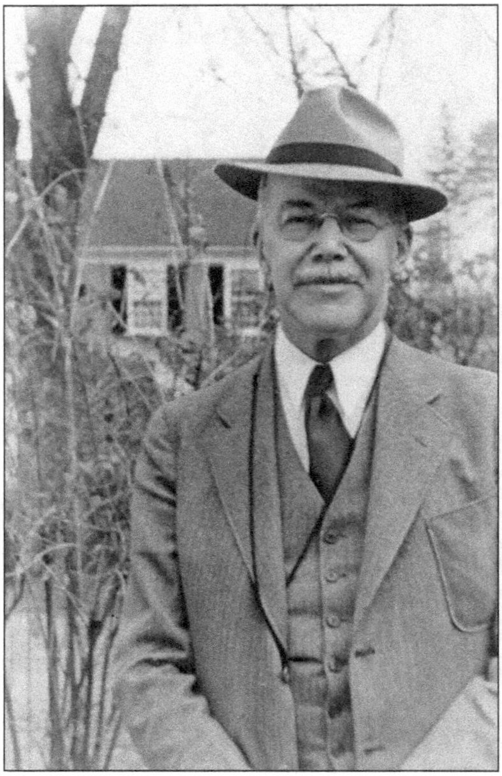

Dr. Charles Wentworth Hoyt, a Boston native and Harvard graduate, was chief of obstetrics, one of the busiest departments. A resident of Main Street in Hingham, he registered for the draft at age 61, along with many other South Shore Hospital physicians. He died a few years after returning from World War II.

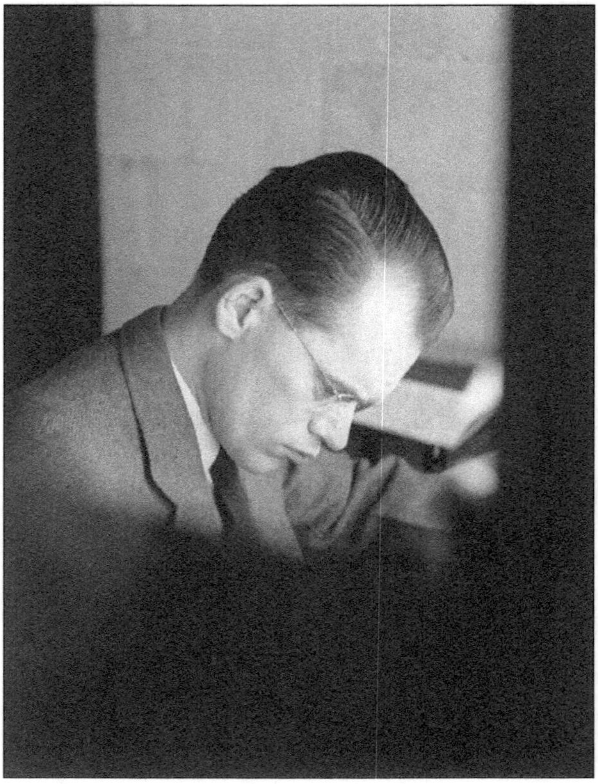

Dr. Folke Wiklund was chief roentgenologist (radiologist) for more than 30 years starting in 1937. His first contract allowed him 40 percent of X-ray fees collected. Unfortunately for him, there were many charity patients plus those who refused to pay. Later, his contract was changed to 33 percent of charges whether paid or not. He created the groundwork for the most proficient radiology department in the region.

Dr. Robert Wilkinson reviews paper prints of X-ray results. From the hospital's earliest days, the ability to see broken bones and tumors within the body was as essential as delivery rooms and operating suites. Donations, like $35,000 from the Archie T. Morrison Foundation and the deep therapy unit from Allan Wheeler given in memory of his in-laws in 1967, helped the hospital upgrade to newer technology.

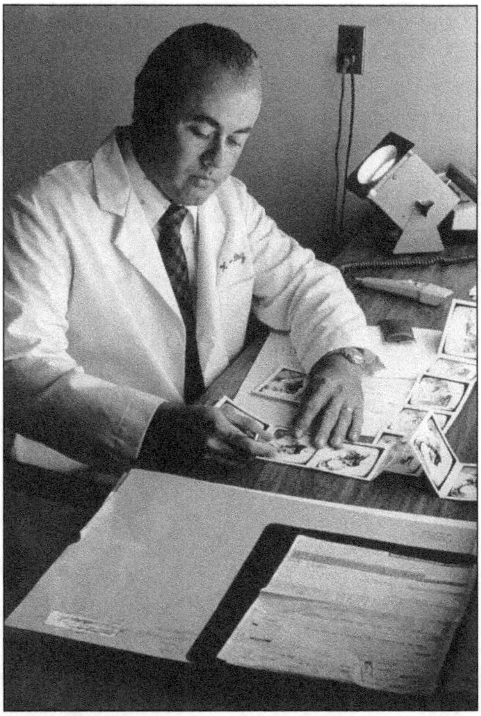

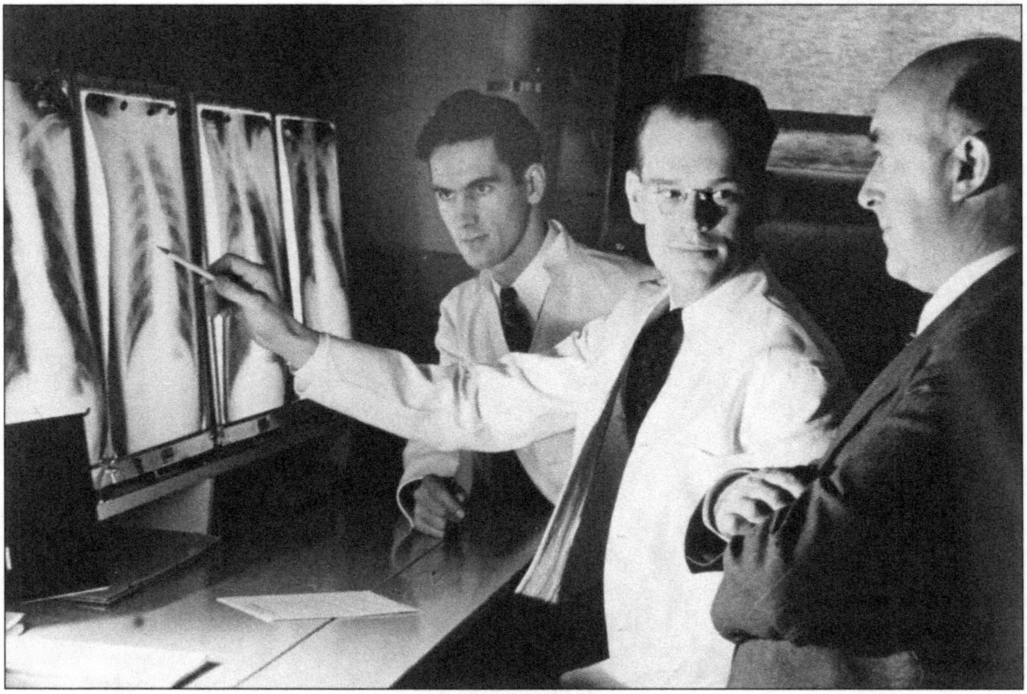

These physicians are likely diagnosing pneumonia. In 1947, patients required 3,884 X-rays and 786 fluoroscopes. In five years, the number increased 25 percent. The department consisted of Dr. Wiklund, the sole roentgenologist, a medical secretary, and three X-ray technicians with two X-ray rooms. Dr. Wiklund and his team continued to produce highly accurate readings despite "working at maximum load in a relatively small department."

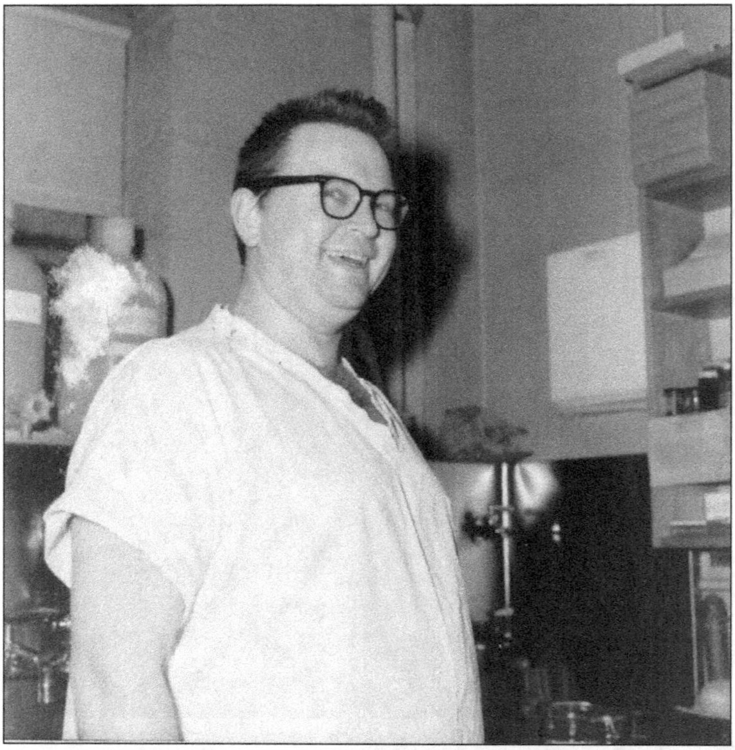

As the hospital grew, the overflow of laboratory examinations was sent to Boston City Hospital. When this arrangement ended in 1958, Dr. John Peters (shown) joined Dr. Pinto in managing the growing laboratory. Peters was medical staff president in 1977. Currently, nearly a million tests are performed annually, and the quality has been recognized repeatedly by national accrediting organizations.

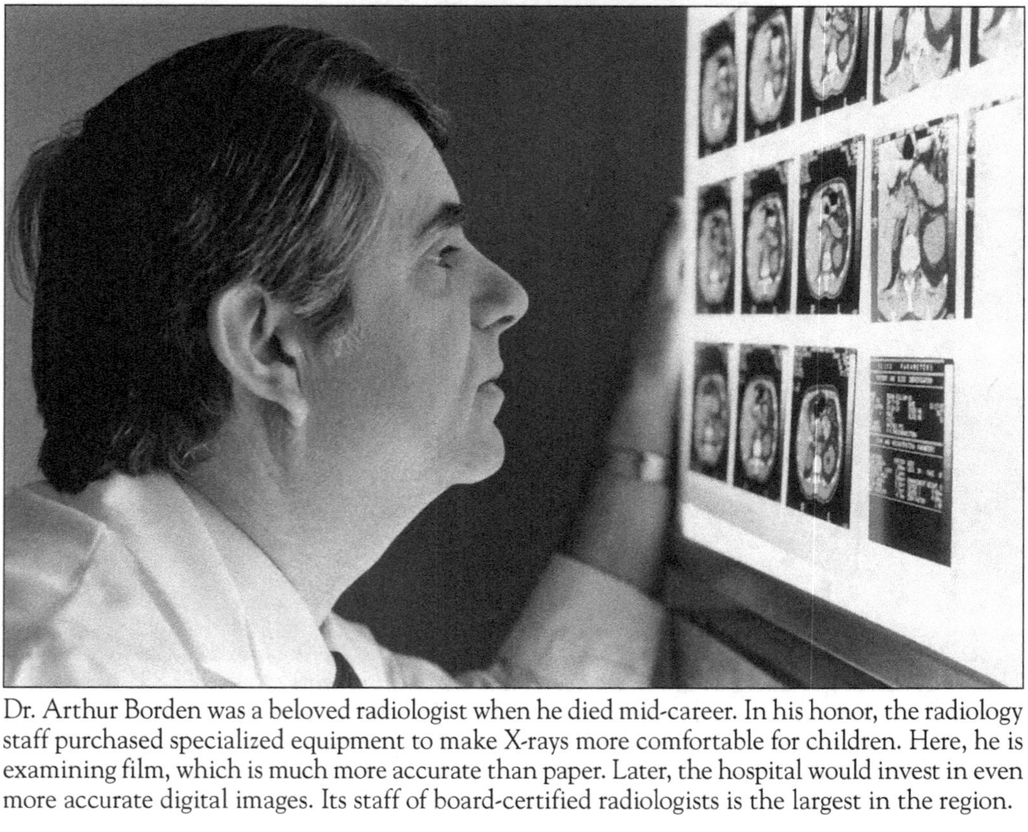

Dr. Arthur Borden was a beloved radiologist when he died mid-career. In his honor, the radiology staff purchased specialized equipment to make X-rays more comfortable for children. Here, he is examining film, which is much more accurate than paper. Later, the hospital would invest in even more accurate digital images. Its staff of board-certified radiologists is the largest in the region.

Dr. James A. Dolphin, of Hingham, joined the medical staff in 1958 and was elected president in 1976. During that year, the top two floors were added to the Laban Pratt building. The Dr. James A. and Mary Lynd Dolphin Surgical Center, including 14 operating rooms with advanced technology and equipment, opened 25 years later.

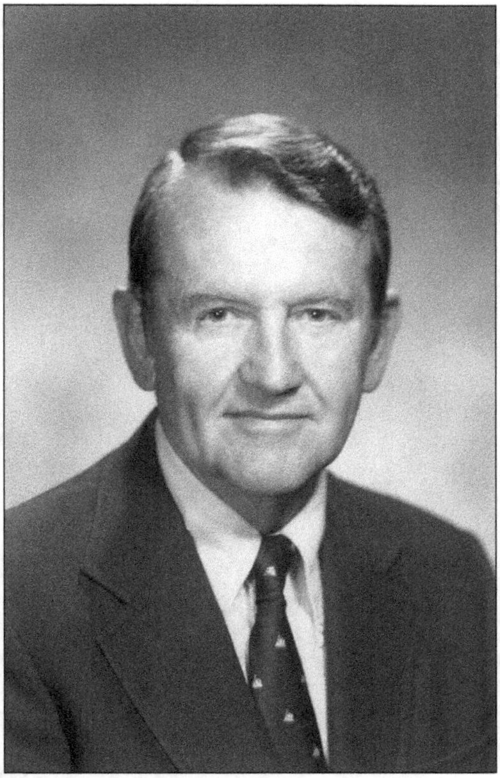

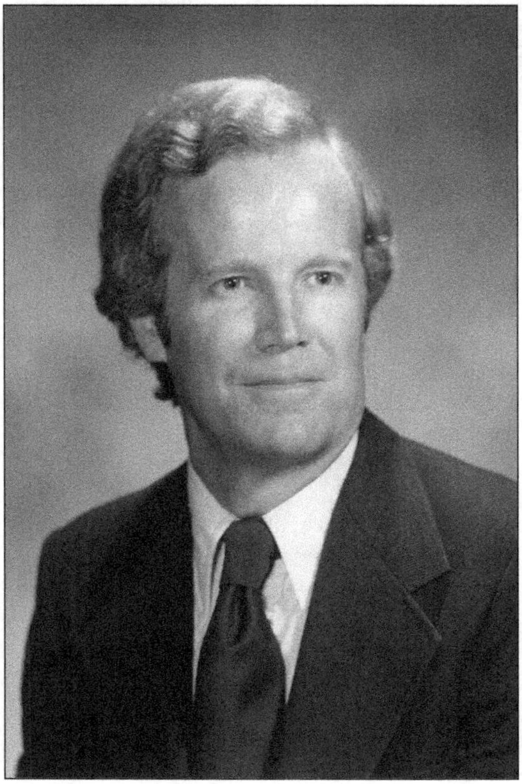

Dr. Paul Duggan was elected medical staff president in 1978. While the majority of physicians come from outside the region, for many, serving is a family tradition. Among the families are Ayers, Cilento, Cox, Duggan, McConville, and Sullivan. The tradition also includes fathers and sons serving as medical staff presidents: Arsham and Richard Alemian, and Edward H. and Edward W. Nalband.

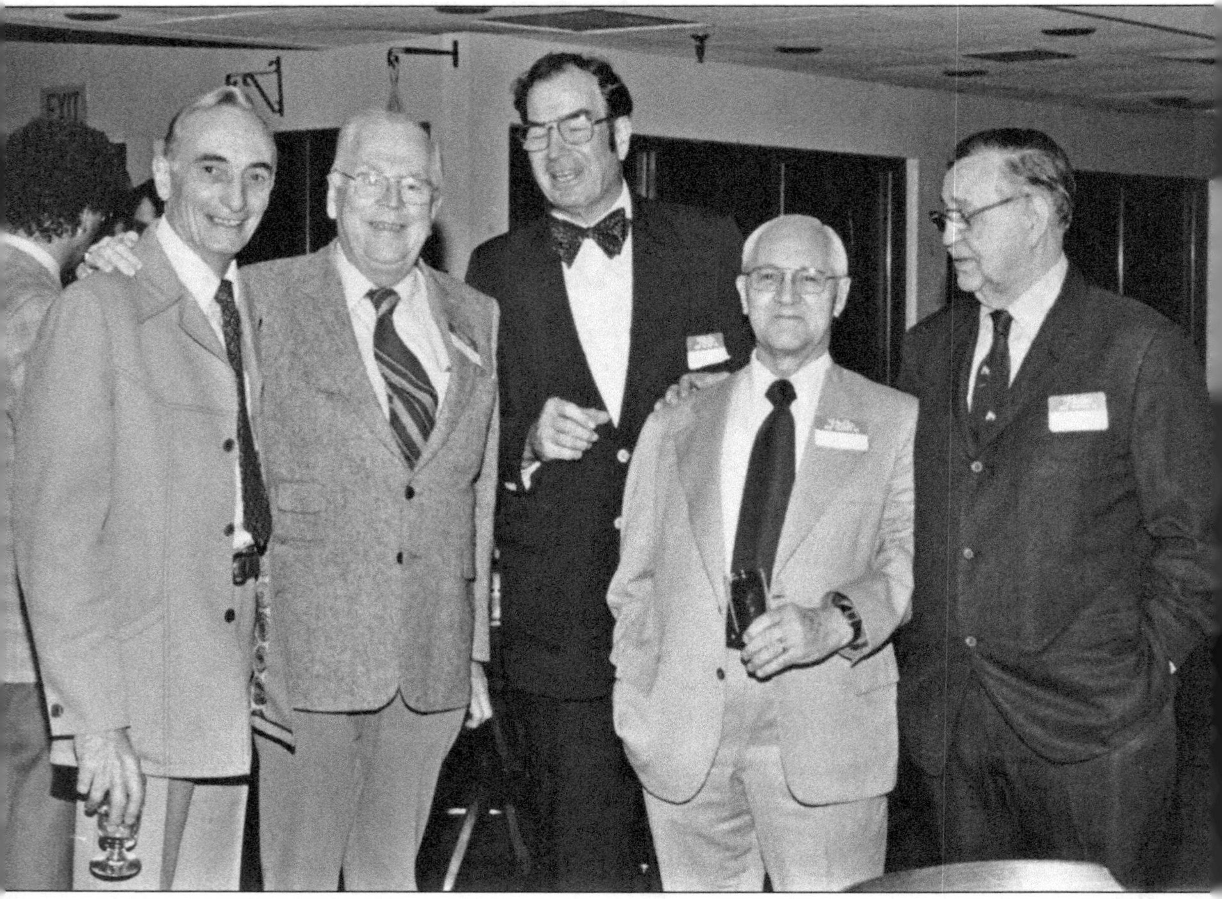

Honoring Dr. Archie Keigan (left), a general practitioner who was medical staff president in 1971, are, from left to right, orthopedic surgeon Dr. Richard Kilfarile and general practitioners Drs. Arthur Sullivan, Frank Durant, and L. Burton Benjamin. Dr. Sullivan's father, Cornelius, along with Drs. Emerson, Doucette, and Drake were the hospital's first medical staff. The bylaws required that the medical board "consist of all the physicians in good standing, resident of and practicing within the Town of Weymouth, and who are members of the Massachusetts Medical Society or like society." Less than 100 years later, the medical staff is the region's largest with more than 900 members, 96 percent board certified in their specialties—well above the Massachusetts average of 74.3 percent. Physicians associated with the hospital have earned leadership positions in medical societies and won recognition for quality care. Once, some Boston physicians doubted that a hospital could survive on the South Shore; now, the hospital's medical staff includes physicians from Brigham and Women's Hospital, Children's Hospital Boston, and Dana-Farber Cancer Institute.

Three

VOLUNTEER LEADERS

PRACTICAL VISIONARIES

The trustees were bold visionaries. In difficult—even dire—financial circumstances, they expanded the hospital when more timid people would have retrenched. They started plans for the $500,000 West Wing when the hospital's funds totaled $15,000, only $1,400 of which was available as cash. They overcame the Depression, global war, nursing shortages, explosive demand for services, anemic insurance reimbursements, and high numbers of charity patients in the early years. With deep roots in Weymouth, they knew precisely what residents needed.

They were compassionate men who felt a personal obligation to care for the less fortunate. They personally covered shortfalls when Blue Cross defaulted on payments. When the hospital could not afford to hire a new superintendent, board president Albert Vinal and trustee Bryan Leonard each gave $800 for three years to supplement his salary.

The trustees managed all nonclinical decisions, checking on everything from the cleanliness of patient rooms to boiler repairs. The hospital was their responsibility.

The years 1944–1945 were a pivotal time for the hospital; it carried a large debt from the 1936 building loan, and reimbursements were far below cost. Operating costs ballooned (postwar food prices increased 75 percent). Vinal, treasurer of the Stetson Shoe Company, restored financial stability. He hired professional managers and persuaded a credit and collections professional to donate his time to reduce overdue accounts. He recruited new trustees. Later, in 2000, the board was streamlined from 27 to 12.

On March 25, 1922, Dr. George E. Emerson, along with William Earle, W. Carleton Barnes, Patrick Derrig, Sidney Dunbar, William Fitzsimmons, William Holbrook, Alonzo Newbert, Parker Pearson, John Reardon, James Smith, and Prince Tirrell, obtained a charter for the Weymouth Hospital. With Earle as president, the first board was comprised of those men plus J. Leonard Bicknell, Arthur Bryant, John Dwyer, Joseph Kelley, Elmer Leonard, Henry Tilden, and Russell Whiting.

Presidents (later called chairmen) of the board were William Earle, W. Carleton Barnes, Florence Hatch, Albert Vinal, Wallace Kemp, E. Curtis Mower, Lawrence Guild, Ervin Hinds, Roy Lawson, George Benedict, Archie Morrison, Donald Shepherd, Stuart Hardy, Shirley Peterson, Richard Swan, Clyde Morrison, and Andrew Gordon.

Also serving as presidents were M. Tucke Curtiss Jr., George Rugman, Sumner Smith Jr., Alan Carr, William Meara Jr., Jane Phillips, Edward Amazeen, Edward McHugh, Harry Healey Jr., Arthur Sharp, James Bristol Jr., David Jones, Paul MacElhiney, Arthur Connelly, Jacqueline Haley, John Doody, Leonard Bicknell, and Brian Hotarek.

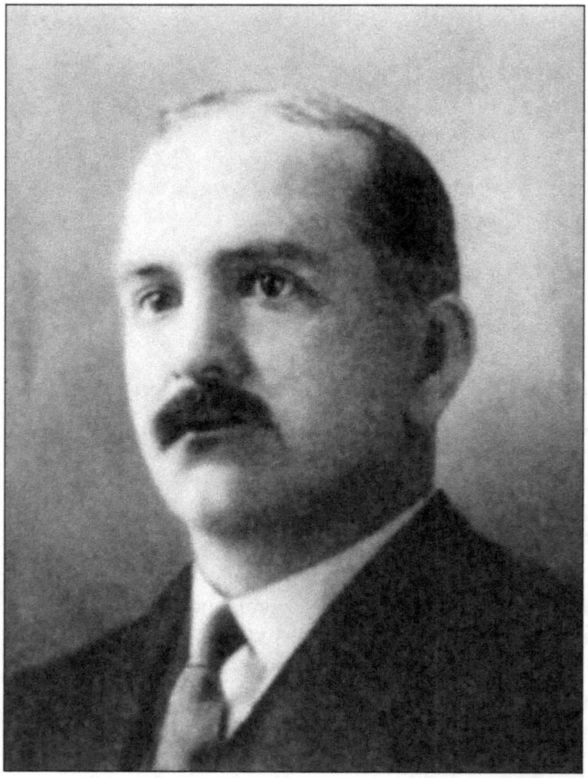

William Earle, 63 (left), was an incorporator and first president of Weymouth Hospital. From East Weymouth, he was custom office deputy surveyor. W. Carleton Barnes (below) was vice president and then president from 1925 until 1943. Barnes, a commercial engineer, obtained the first Public Works Administration funding ever for the Administration Building. For Barnes and his wife Alice, the hospital was their family. She devoted thousands of volunteer hours. They established a library in memory of their son Willard in 1936 and stocked it with 600 of their own books. During World War II, Barnes grew frustrated as "more Bureaus, Committees and Minor Officials have to be consulted with the resulting delays" on the Center Building. Overseeing the hospital worsened his health. He sent copious typed notes to the board from home. He died in 1944, before work began on the building.

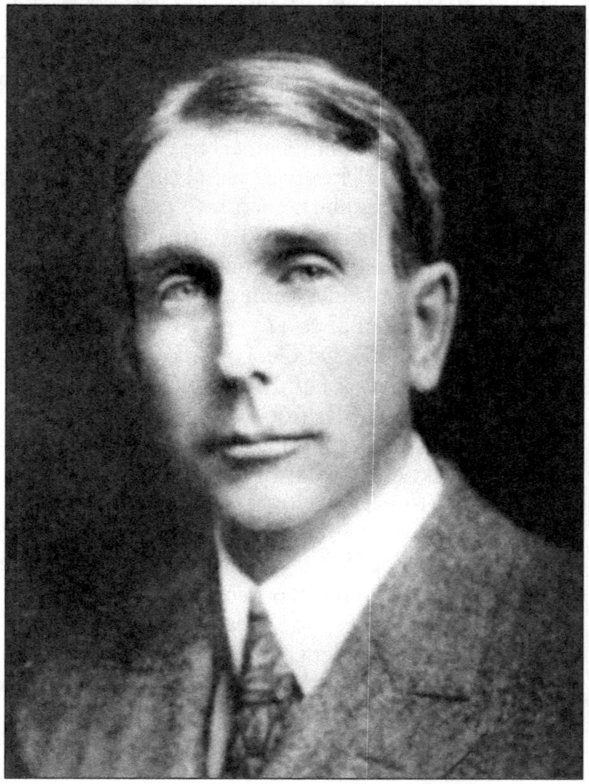

Donald Shepherd (board president from 1960 to 1962) designed a pension system in 1969, which nearly all employees joined. Loyalty expressed through longevity was commonplace. In his report to the board, he noted that employees continued to work even after they qualified for pensions. Part-time employees started to accrue vacation time. In 1970, there were 800 employees.

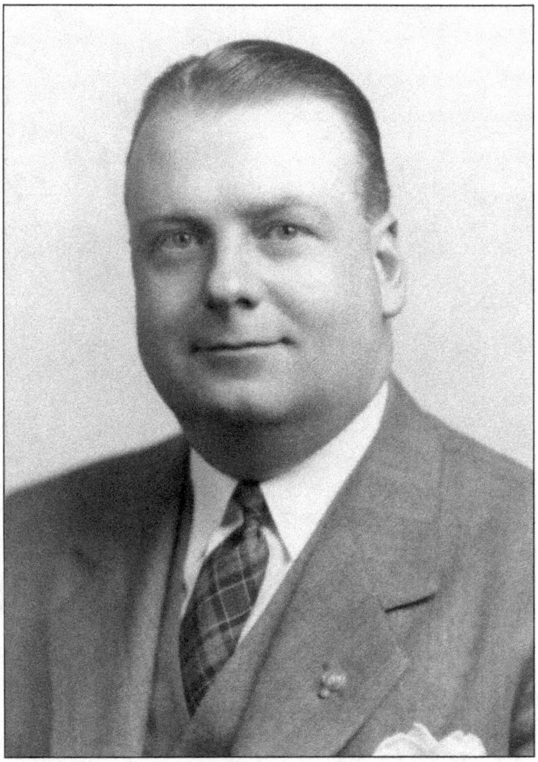

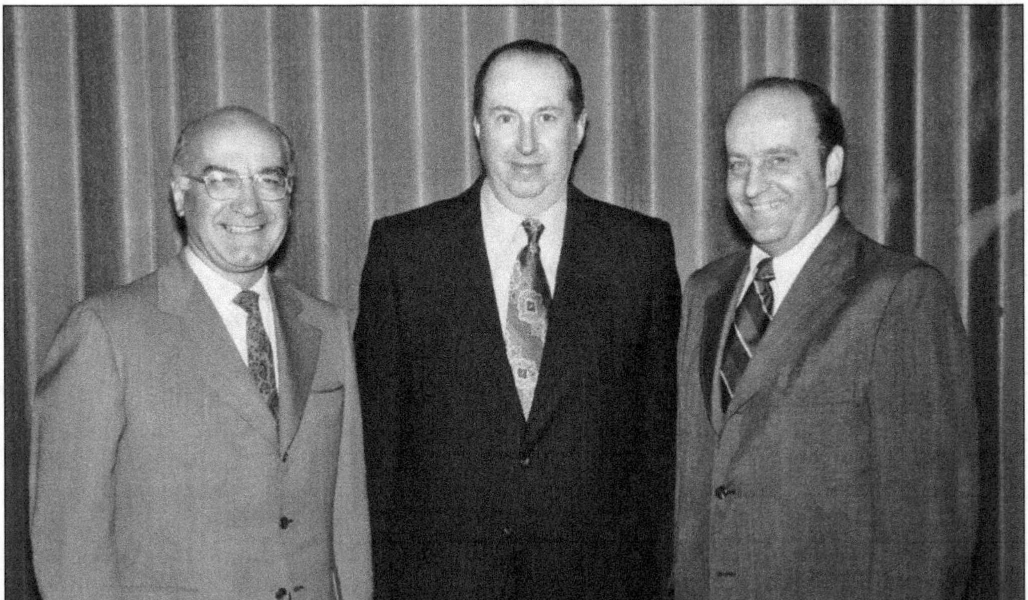

From left to right, medical staff president Dr. Edward Nalband, board chairman George Rugman, and hospital president William Clark had good reason to smile in 1973. The hospital once again pioneered several innovations: one of the nation's first unit-dose systems for medications, and family-centered maternity care with prepared childbirth classes and sibling visiting privileges, then one of only 22 such programs nationwide.

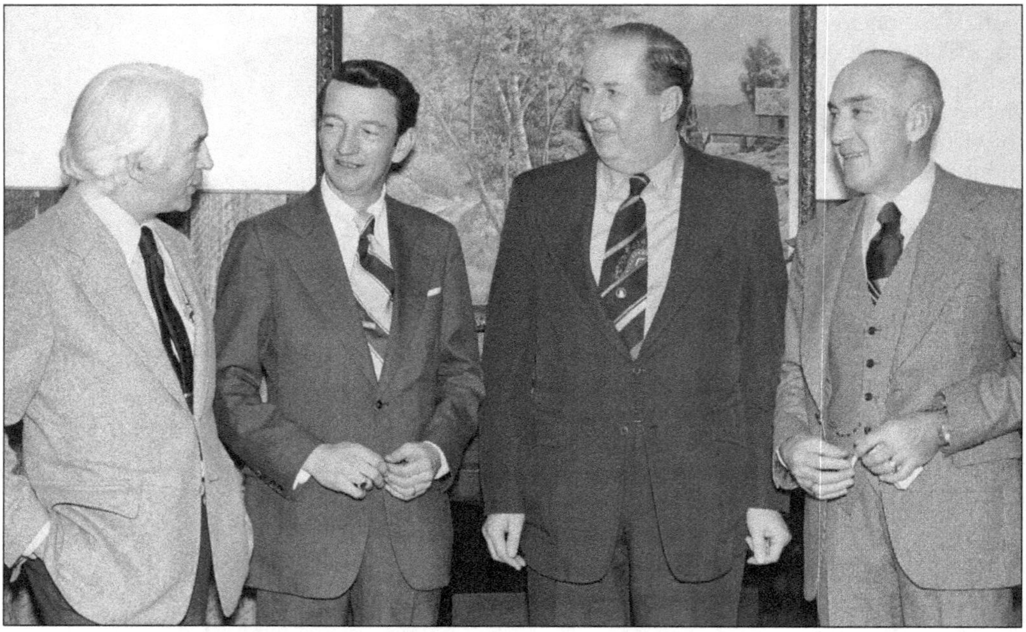

In the 1970s and 1980s, the hospital reorganized its corporate structure and governance. Board members leading the changes in 1979 are, from left to right, Sumner Smith Jr., Alan Carr, George Rugman, and William Meara. In 1982, South Shore Health and Educational Corporation, the new not-for-profit charitable parent corporation, was created to oversee South Shore Hospital and other subsidiaries.

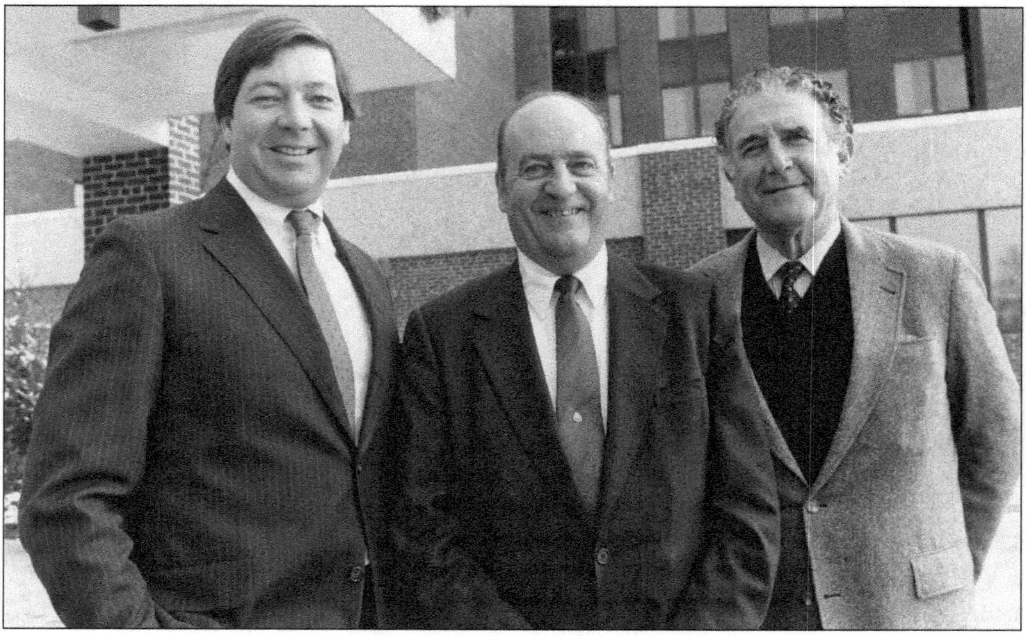

In this 1985 photograph, board chair Edward Amazeen (left) with advice from president William Clark (center) and medical staff president Dr. Albert Marcus, created South Shore Properties, a corporate subsidiary. It developed the Nevin Professional Building, medical condominiums on Main Street that brought the physicians closer to the Weymouth Campus. The hospital also introduced an organization-wide computer system and acquired a full-body CT scanner.

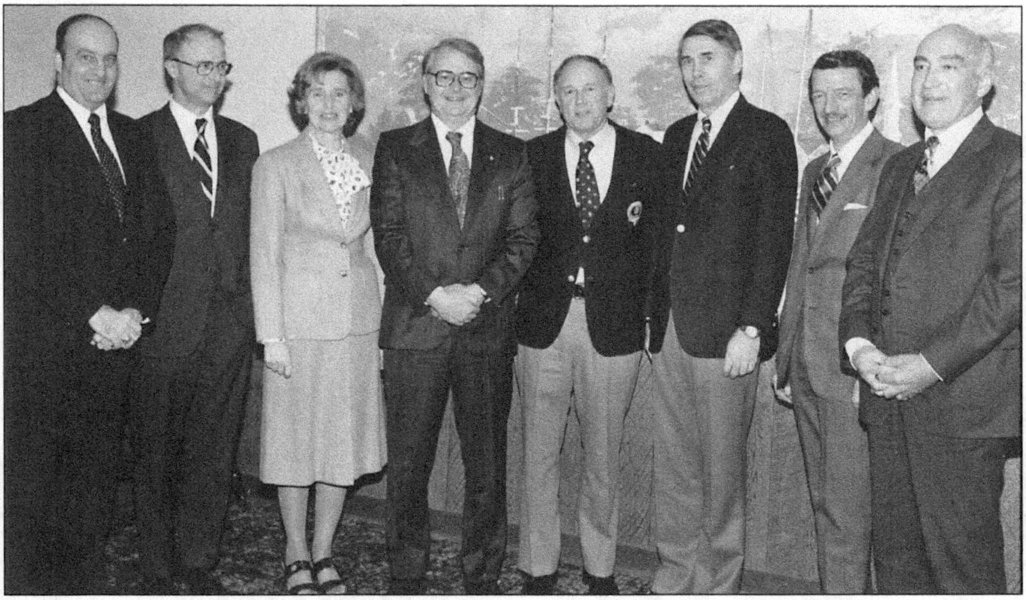

Hospital president William Clark retired after 17 years. A decade of hospital leaders offered their congratulations. With dates of chairmanship in parenthesis are, from left to right, Clark, Edward McHugh (1985–1986), Jane Phillips (1983–1984), Harry Healey (1988–1989), M. Tucke Curtiss (1973–1974), and Directors David Chase, Alan Carr (1979–1980), and William F. Meara Jr. (1980–1982). During their collective tenures, the hospital opened the Laban Pratt and Chassis Buildings to serve thousands more patients annually.

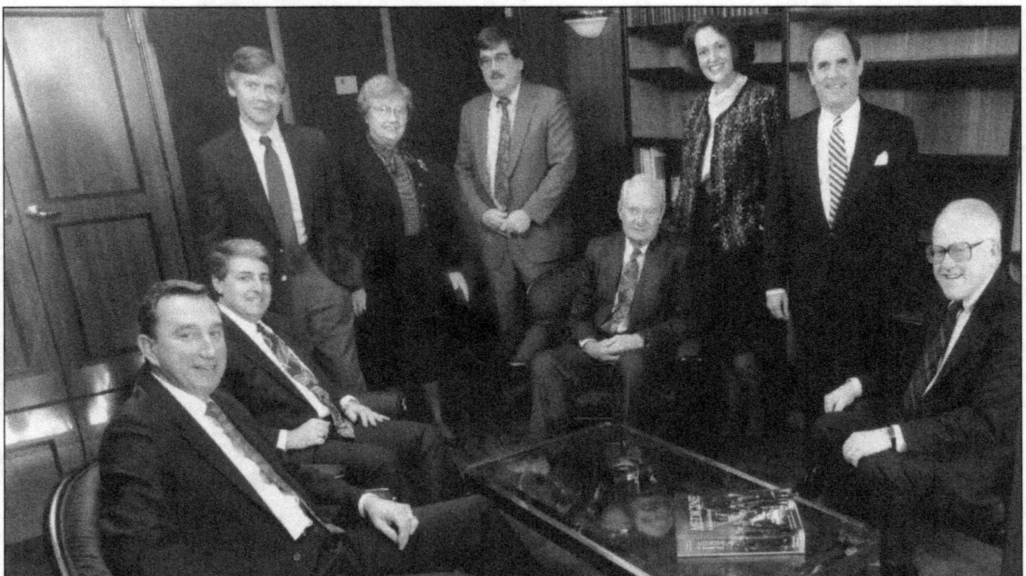

Hospital leaders in 1991 are, from left to right, Arthur Sharp, chairman; Steven Marini, South Shore Visiting Nurse Association (VNA) board chairman; Dr. James Penza, medical staff president; Barbara Hamer, Friends of South Shore Hospital president; George Laban, VNA president; C. Herbert Emilson, South Shore Health & Educational Foundation (now South Shore Hospital Charitable Foundation) board chairman; Patricia Pomerleau, executive vice president; David Hannan, president and chief executive officer; and Harry Healey Jr., chairman.

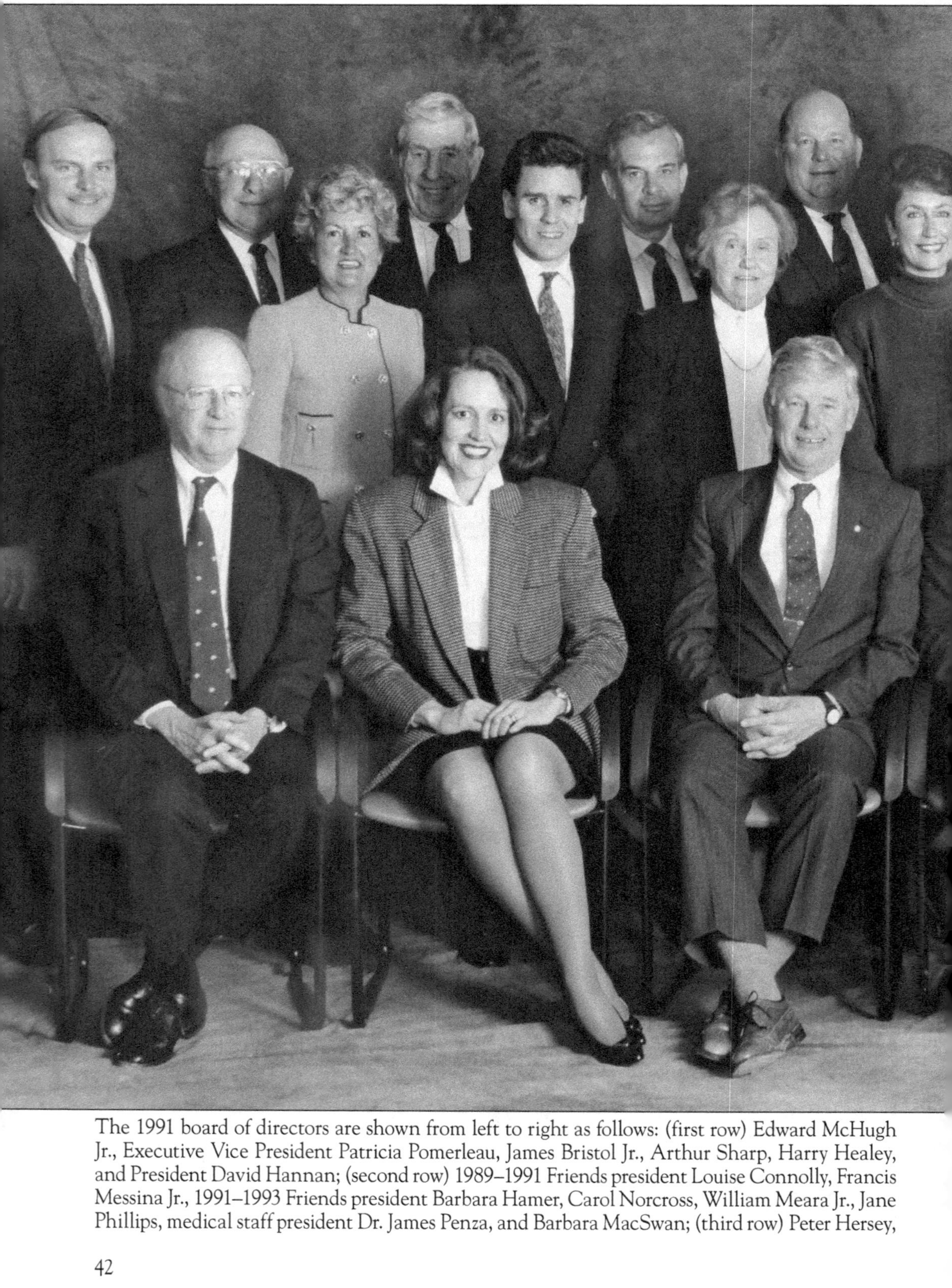

The 1991 board of directors are shown from left to right as follows: (first row) Edward McHugh Jr., Executive Vice President Patricia Pomerleau, James Bristol Jr., Arthur Sharp, Harry Healey, and President David Hannan; (second row) 1989–1991 Friends president Louise Connolly, Francis Messina Jr., 1991–1993 Friends president Barbara Hamer, Carol Norcross, William Meara Jr., Jane Phillips, medical staff president Dr. James Penza, and Barbara MacSwan; (third row) Peter Hersey,

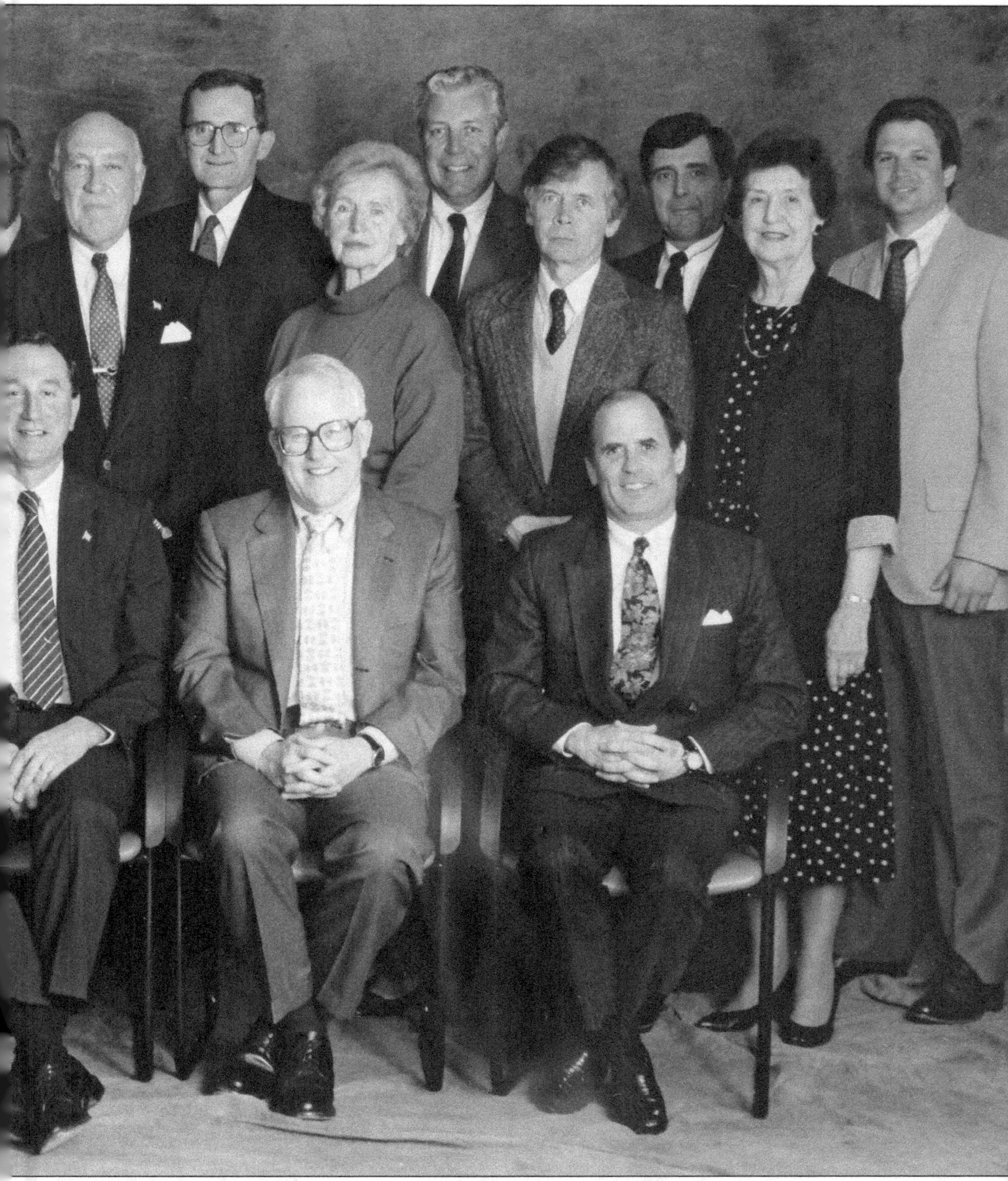

Louis Cataldo, Ernest Minelli Jr., Dr. Philip Landry, Donald Olson, Dr. Richard Alemian, Dr. Frederick Ayers, Paul MacElhiney, C. Alan Chambers, and Preston Hoffman. The hospital was the first in Massachusetts to earn the maximum three-year accreditation with commendation from the Joint Commission on Accreditation of Healthcare Organizations (now the Joint Commission). It grew from the 18th to 10th busiest acute care hospital in Massachusetts between the late 1980s and 1992.

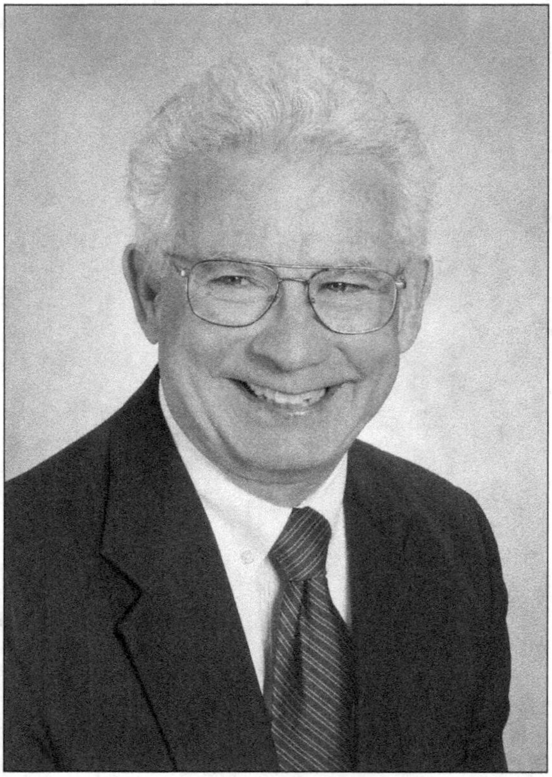

John C. Doody was a member and chairman of South Shore Hospital Charitable Foundation board of trustees, chairman of the Heart of the South Shore capital campaign, and a member and chairman of South Shore Hospital board. He was named an honorary board chair and trustee emeritus by both the hospital and Foundation boards.

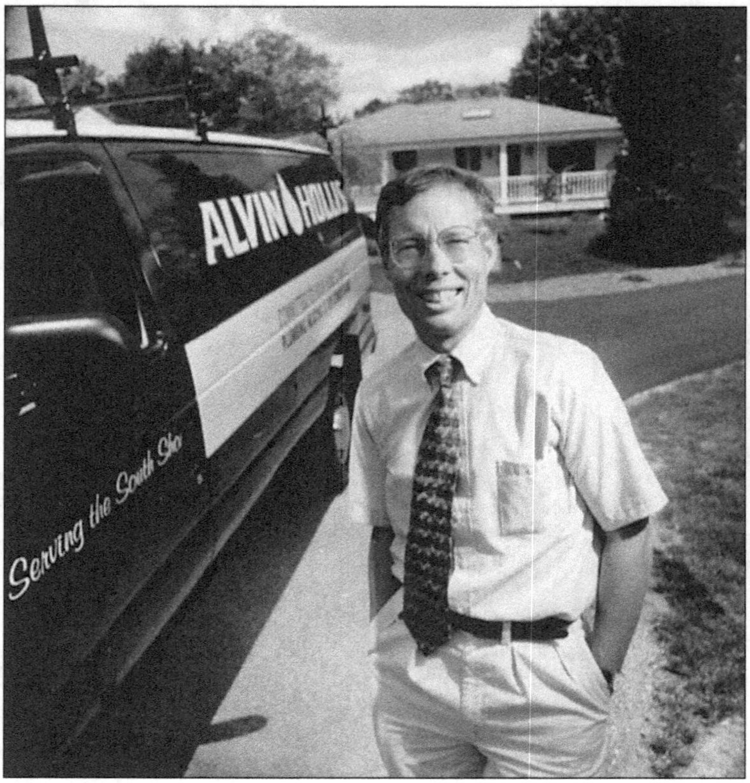

J. Leonard Bicknell, president of Alvin Hollis Company in South Weymouth, was a member of both the hospital and Foundation boards. His mother, Gertrude, was a South Shore Hospital nurse when she cared for Alvin Bicknell, who she would later marry. Alvin also became a hospital board member. Along with their many charitable efforts, Leonard's wife, Dolly, and daughter Laura led the annual Walk for Hospice.

Four

Colleagues and Staff

Creating a Culture of Caring

From its earliest days with a staff of less than 20, South Shore Hospital has grown to one of the largest non-government employers in southeastern Massachusetts with a workforce of 3,800. The staff has grown more professional with 1,500 registered nurses. Unlike many hospitals, South Shore Hospital refuses to allow nursing care to be provided by unlicensed caregivers.

Leading the hospital have been supervisors Irene Estabrook Oliver and Kate Blandford, Directors Dr. Arthur Perkins and Donald Duke, and Presidents William Clark, David Hannan, and Richard Aubut. Until Dr. Perkins arrived, the trustees made all nonclinical decisions, ranging from hiring staff to buying supplies.

The staff's professionalism and expertise have been recognized at the highest levels. The Joint Commission has consistently rated the hospital in the top tier nationally. The hospital received one of its most significant honors from the American Nurses Credentialing Center, which awarded its coveted Magnet Status for excellence in nursing. Only seven percent of all hospitals nationwide have achieved this honor.

President Richard Aubut described the hospital's culture of caring: "We recognize the outstanding work by our nurses each day in caring for their patients and each other. This reflects the commitment of our entire staff to serve as a team, providing the highest quality care possible for the people of our community."

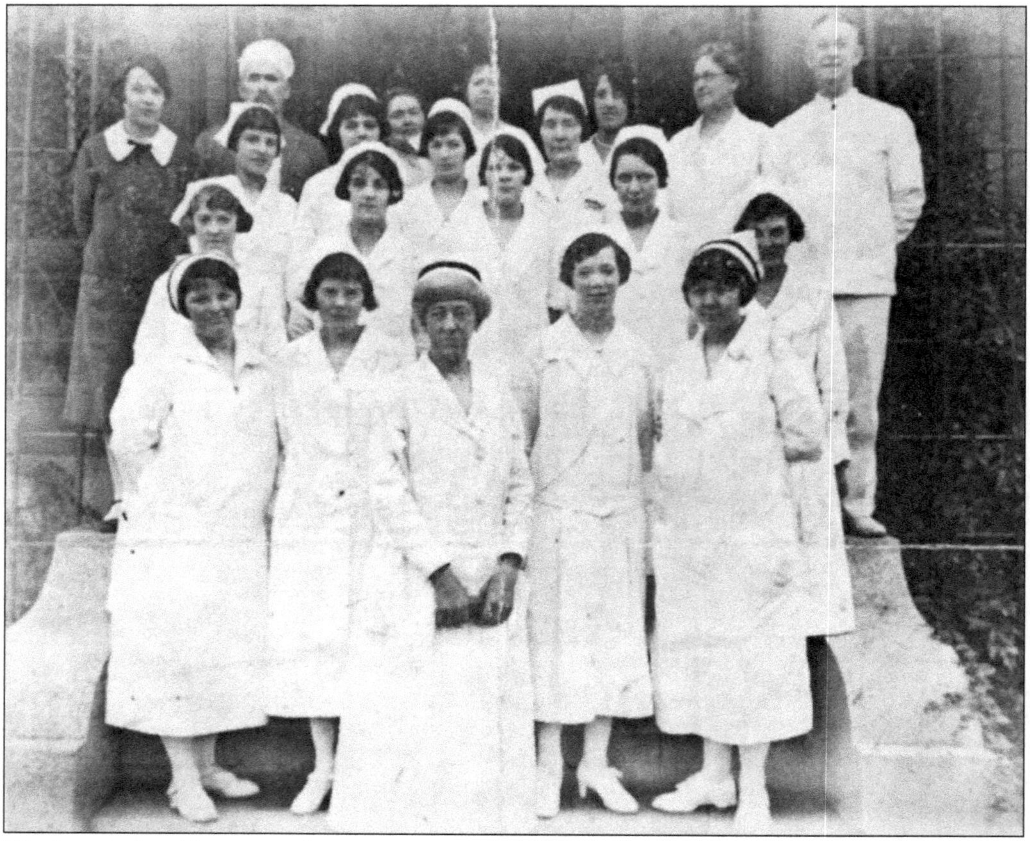

The hospital staff poses at the entrance in 1926. The hospital continued to provide room and board to nurses for a fee. In 1949, the hospital agreed to end the practice of deducting room and board from nurses' salaries and to substitute cash payments instead. Homes bordering the campus were purchased for nurses' residences until the late 1950s.

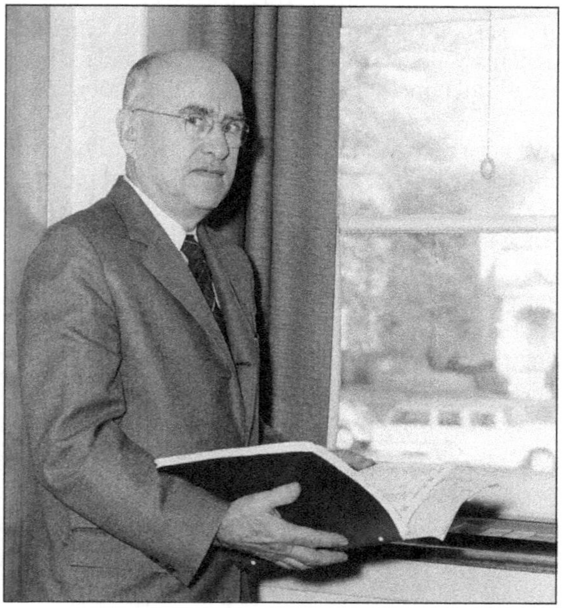

Dr. Arthur E. Perkins was the hospital's first administrator. A physician experienced in hospital administration, he arrived in January 1945 amid the move into a new building. Perkins inspired through his "gentleness under his apparently stern demeanor, [and] his very definite concept of what a good community hospital should offer its patients."

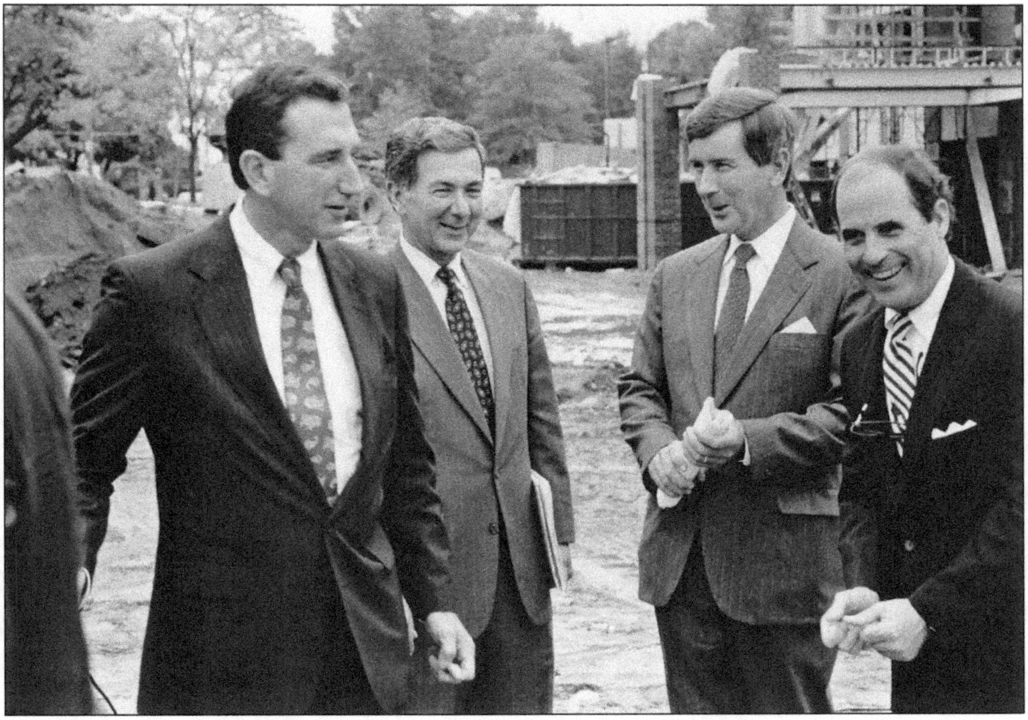

Donald Duke and William Clark succeeded Perkins. In 1986, Clark retired after 17 years, and David Hannan was elected president and chief executive officer. During Hannan's 17-year tenure, the hospital established its preeminence, added over $100 million in new buildings, and won numerous awards for quality. Hannan (right) greets, from left, Director Arthur Sharp, New England Medical Center president Richard Nesson, and television news personality Peter Mehegan at the Emerson Building dedication.

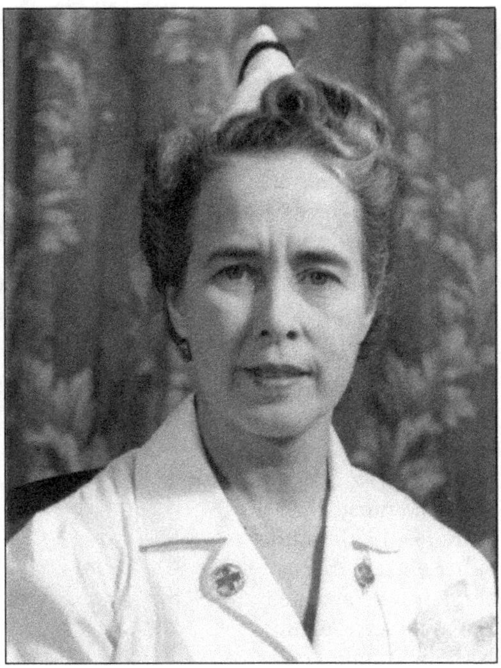

Irene Estabrook Oliver was appointed superintendent in 1930 and led the hospital during the Depression and the nursing shortages of World War II. She was a fulcrum between the staff and the keenly involved volunteer board. She tended her resignation in 1943 when Carleton Barnes resigned as president, but the trustees declined it, accepting it a year later with gratitude for her accomplishments.

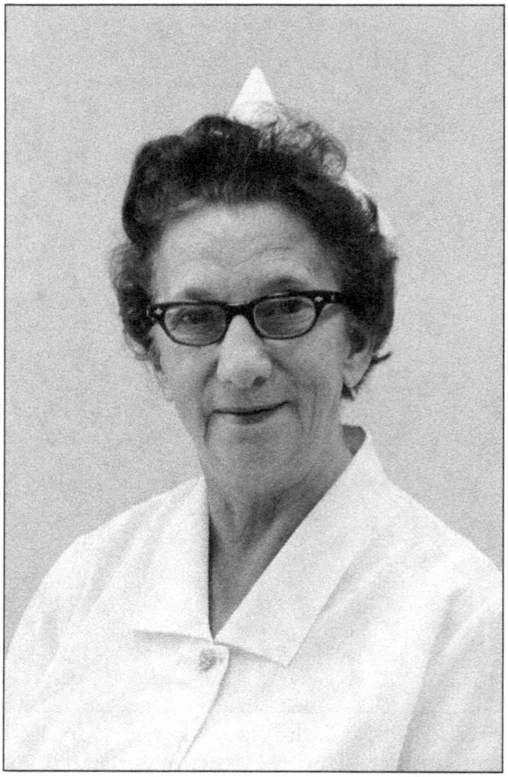

Kate Blandford was director of nursing for 25 years, succeeding Oliver. She would find creative ways to overcome the shortage of nurses, including hiring young nurses to work part-time around family obligations. When she retired in 1968, trustee Henry Hoffman said, "The high morale of the nursing staff was due to the leadership of Miss Blandford."

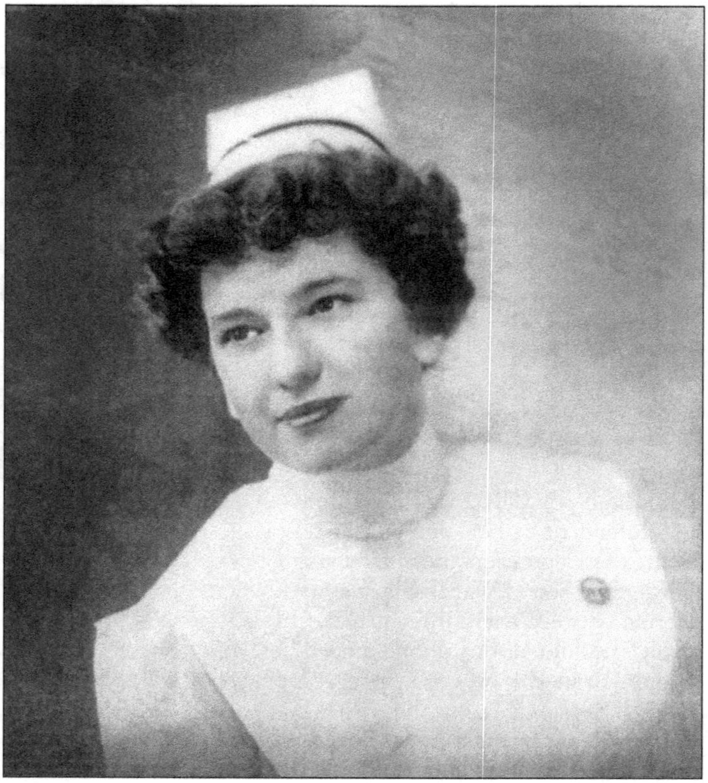

Therese Yvonne Boucher Ries, a Canadian nurse, came to America as a private-duty nurse for a Weymouth couple injured in a car accident. While raising her family, she worked in the first "accident room" in the Center Building. As emergency and trauma services expanded, she was head nurse until she retired in 1970. In honor of her 48-year career, her family established a nursing scholarship at the hospital.

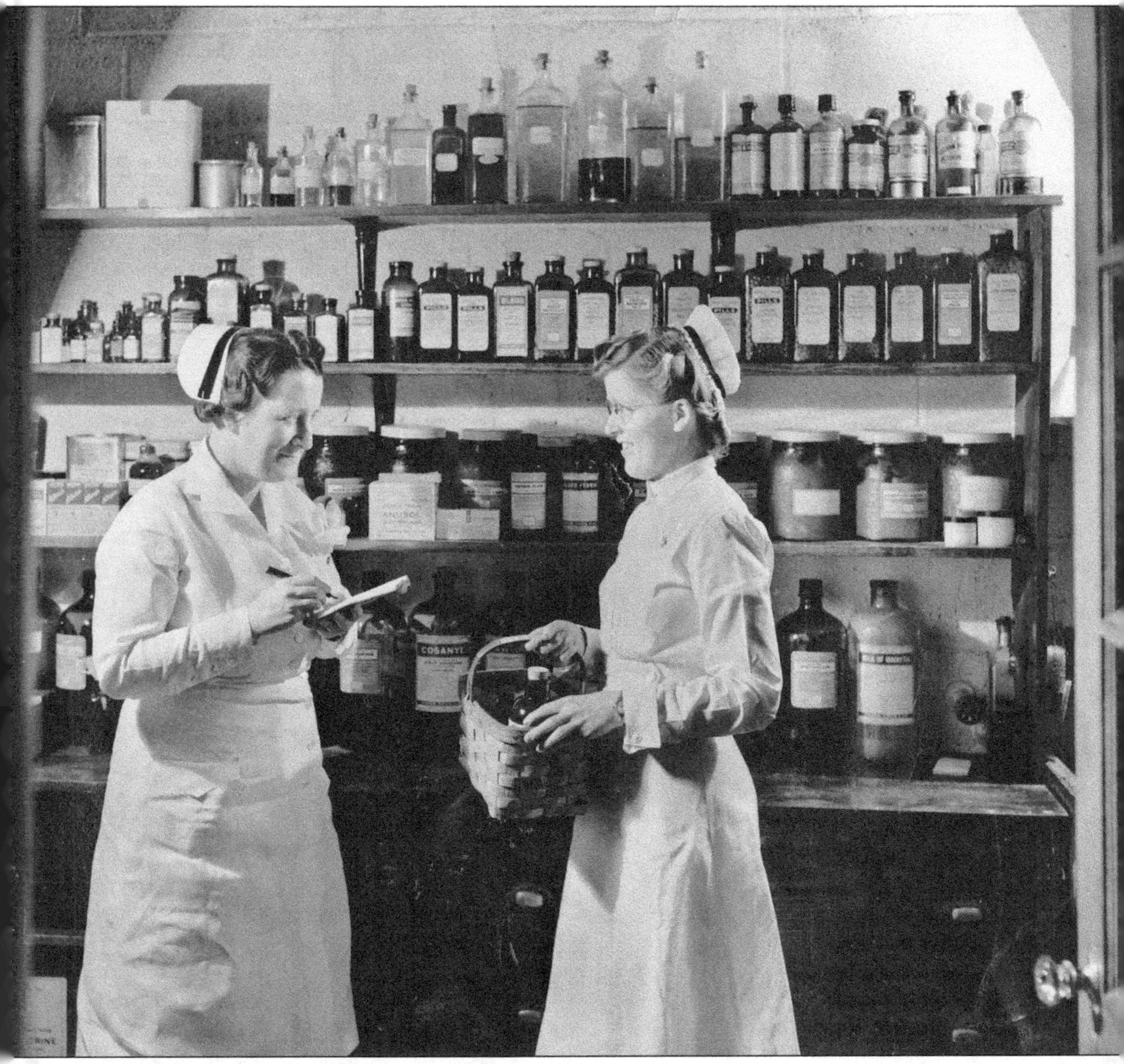

In the 1930s and 1940s, nurses regularly prepared medication doses. Often, liquid medications were stored in cork-top bottles with handwritten labels. Nurses used step stools to reach medications on upper shelves and had to be vigilant that they chose the right bottle. In this photograph, nurse Mary Morrissey (left) maintains the inventory while nurse Grace Hurley prepares to deliver medications in a wicker basket. Morrissey wears an open-neck-collar shirtdress with an elaborate handkerchief. Hurley's starched uniform features a high collar, French-cuff shirt, and a high-waisted skirt. Instead of a handkerchief, she proudly displays her nursing pin. The hospital now utilizes sophisticated systems loaded with safeguards to ensure that patients receive the right medications, in the correct doses, and on time. The pharmacy employs professional pharmacists to prepare doses that are double-checked and usually dispensed by computers.

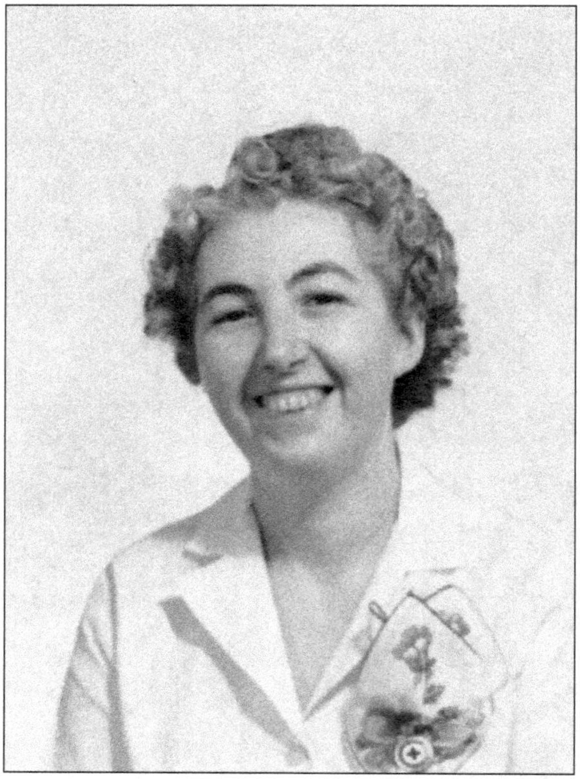

Pearl Hastay was chief admitting officer in 1954 when this photograph was taken. That year, 6,418 patients received care. Before and during construction of the West Wing, Hastay had to locate beds in a hospital with a high occupancy rate while whole departments were moved. Even after the building opened, 300 patients awaited admission.

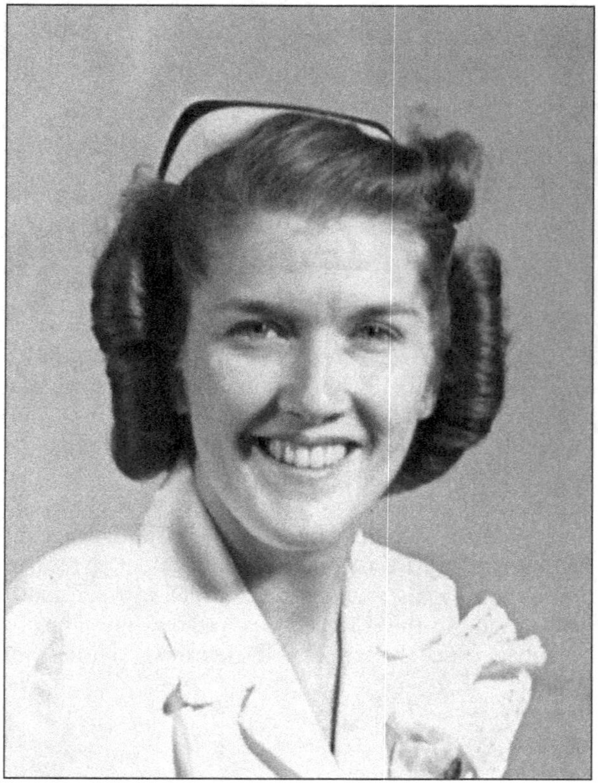

Despite a severe shortage of skilled nurses, caregivers like Dorothy Curtin assured that patients received excellent care. After the severe shortages during and after World War II, the nursing staff finally stabilized in 1953. Turnover was down to 25 percent, the lowest since before World War II. However, private-duty nurses continued to be in great demand.

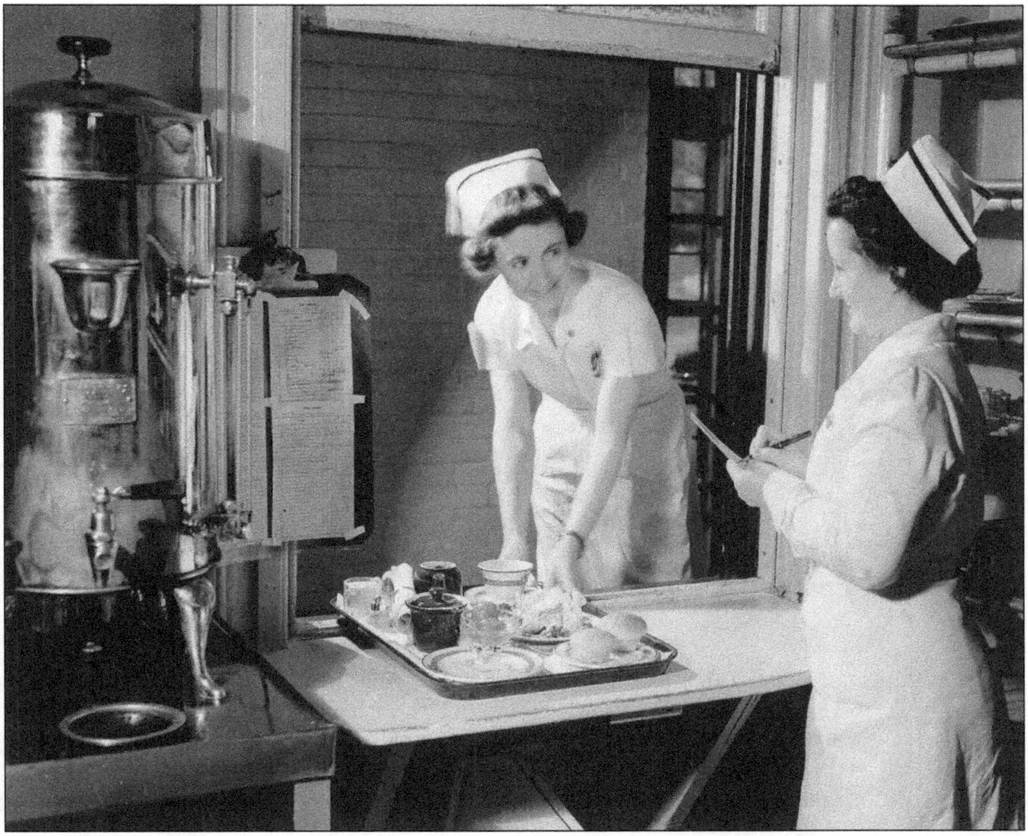

Above, Adelaide Smith (right) checks the food tray for an unidentified nurse. In 1948, the nurses tracked all meals and dietary restrictions for the 4,400 patients by hand. Coffee was prepared in great samovars, and meals were served on heavy china presented on linen hand sewn by the Women's Guild. After the war, the guild was replaced by the Friends of South Shore Hospital, which continued to sew table linens and other items to make patients' stays more comfortable. The cost of preparing meals soared in 1948. Hospital president W. Curtiss Mower wrote that the hospital's per-meal raw food cost increased 75 percent in less than three years—from 29¢ to 51¢. The total cost of food was $91,540 in 1948. Annual reports listed urgently needed items. Among them were teapots ($4.30), Waring blenders ($40), and a dish-washing machine ($2,500). At right is a photograph of a typical meal tray, dressed with individual glass salt-and-pepper shakers.

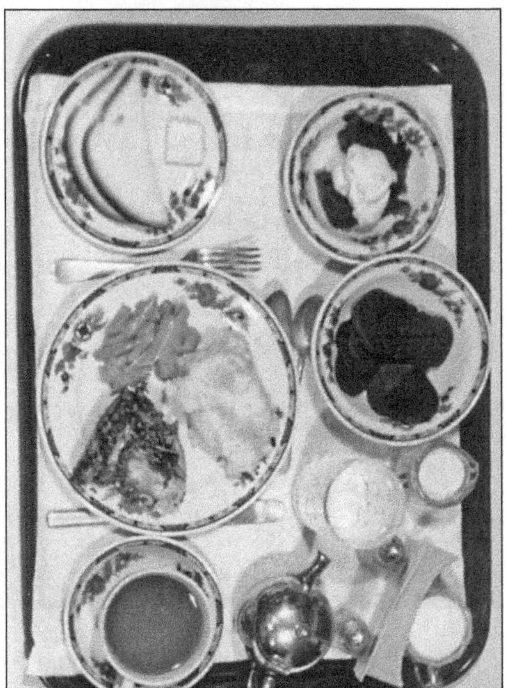

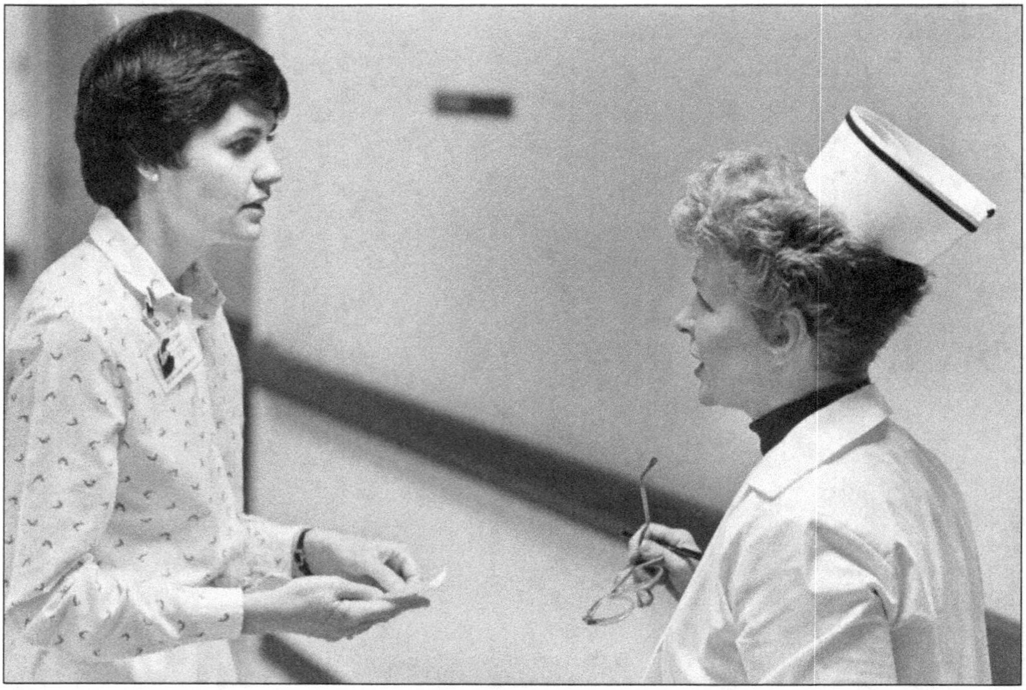

As South Shore Hospital grew, the need for more nurses with specialized expertise increased. Mary Ellen Concannon (left), the hospital's first oncology nurse, confers with nursing supervisor Elizabeth McCarthy Ezekiel. For those patients who no longer benefited from aggressive medical services, the hospital provided the region's first hospice and palliative care.

Until the late 1980s, the hospital's logotype was a stylized rod of Asclepius and lamp of learning. This pin commemorates the 50th anniversary in 1972. Through the Depression, unprecedented population growth, financial constraints, and the hospital's expansion, the staff grew more skilled, more organized, and more committed. The pin was a badge of honor.

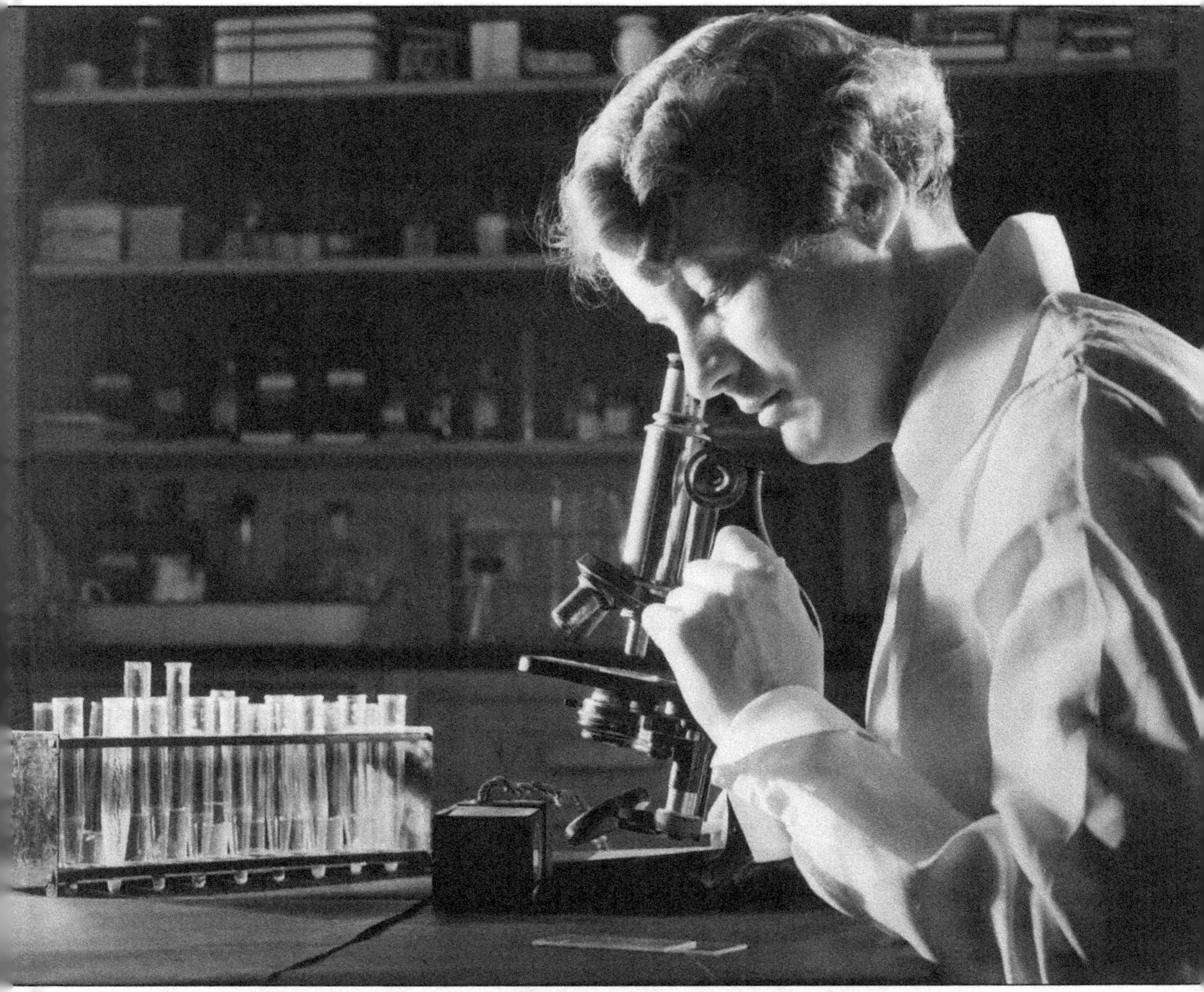

Edith Smith was the hospital's first laboratory technician in 1932. She remained its mainstay for decades. She described the hospital during the war years: "In that first laboratory, we had a cot for patients who had to lie down but the hospital was always stuffed full. It grieved them to see that empty bed in my anteroom, so they used to put patients in there. . . . Everyone was always busy. . . . I worked in the accident room. I gave anesthesia. I did X-ray and the lab. I used to admit and discharge patients, figure up the bills, and run the switchboard. Anything that needed to be done, we all did it." In 1967, she was chief technologist with additional responsibilities for daily operations. By then, the laboratory handled 114,000 tests. The laboratory's accuracy and efficiency was largely due to her experience and high standards.

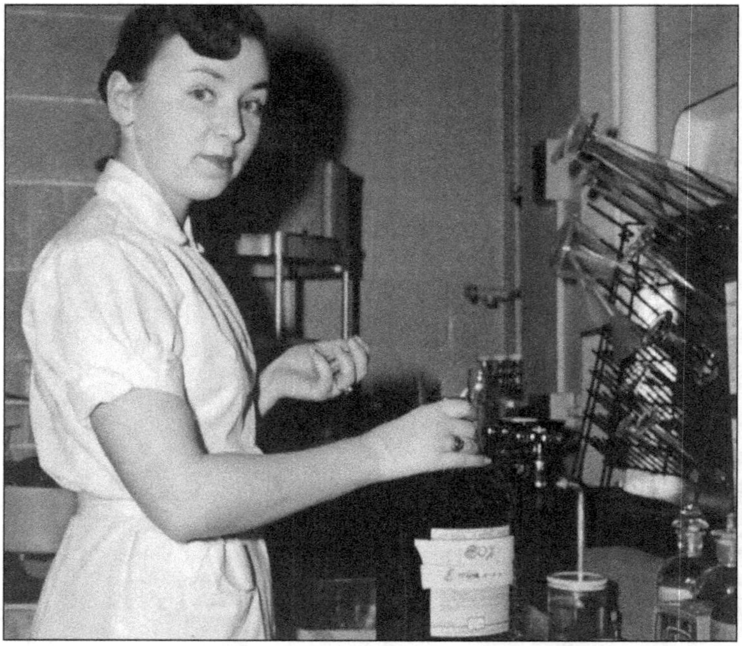

Jacqueline Booth and Dwayne Lancaster prepare samples in the newly expanded laboratory. In 1948, the laboratory's new quarters in the Center Building were double the size of the Administration Building laboratory. With more people moving to suburbia, the staff produced increasing numbers of examinations and autopsies. Between 1948 and 1952, examinations nearly doubled, but the staff remained rigorously accurate, due to Edith Smith's quality control. Although considered modern at the time, the laboratory lacked modern air filtering and sterile conditions. Staff lacked bench space to add and test much-needed new equipment, and some of its existing instruments were described as "delicate, capricious, and temperamental." Director Dr. John Peters wrote, "The laboratory is not a gadget into which specimens go and results come out. The laboratory is the result of the hard work, conscientiousness, interest, integrity and devotion of the people in it."

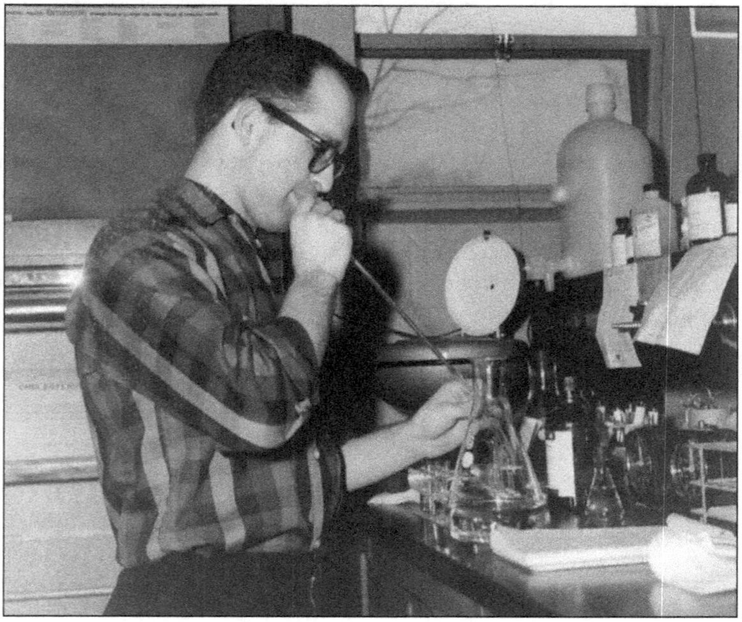

John Vining, laboratory assistant, built and repaired equipment in the laboratory's workshop and ran tests on tissue samples. When the Administration Building was completed in 1936, the laboratory moved from the mansion into rooms where sterilized equipment could be maintained. By 1948, the staff completed 25,000 examinations. They also performed 24 autopsies, about 16 percent of all deaths at the hospital. J. Stewart Rooney, of Boston, was the pathologist.

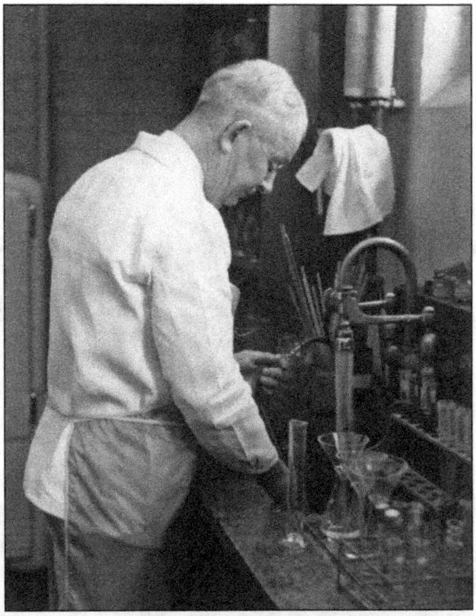

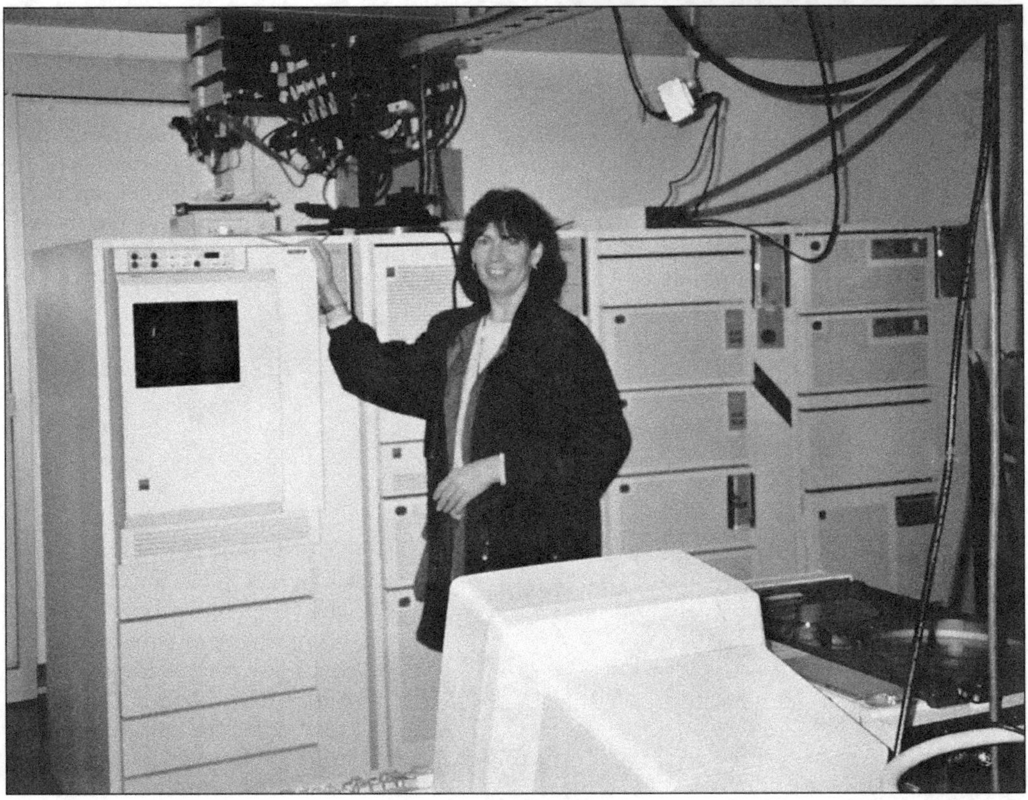

Until the first computers were introduced in the 1960s, hours worked by staff were tallied by hand in ledgers. In 1989, Patrice Lynch Perrotta demonstrates the hospital's newest investment, an IBM AS/400 system, equivalent to three desktop computers today. The hospital's current state-of-the-art information systems center houses 254 servers and three storage-area networks with about 100 terabytes and multiple firewalls for security.

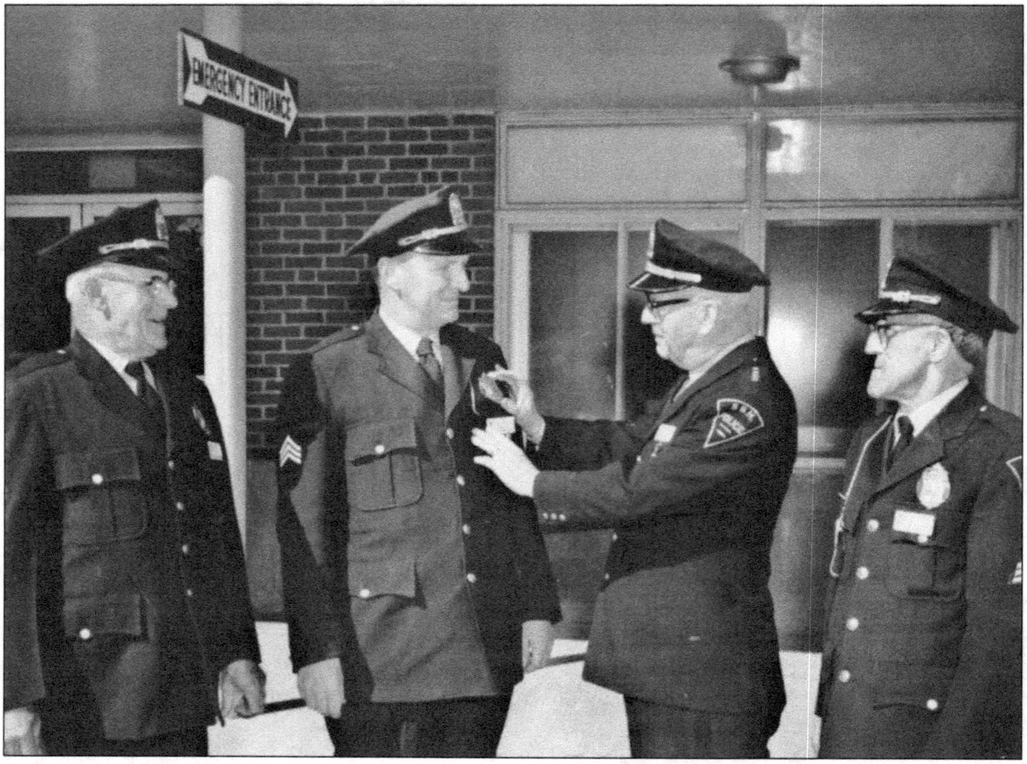

Edward Cahill (second from left) receives his badge to join the hospital's security team from Chief John Coyle. The unit formed in 1967 with six uniformed officers: a chief, two officers, and three night watchers, all appointed as special police officers by the Board of Selectmen of Weymouth. Currently, the 30-member public safety department is responsible for the security of a multi-campus setting and hundreds of thousands of patients, families, visitors, and staff.

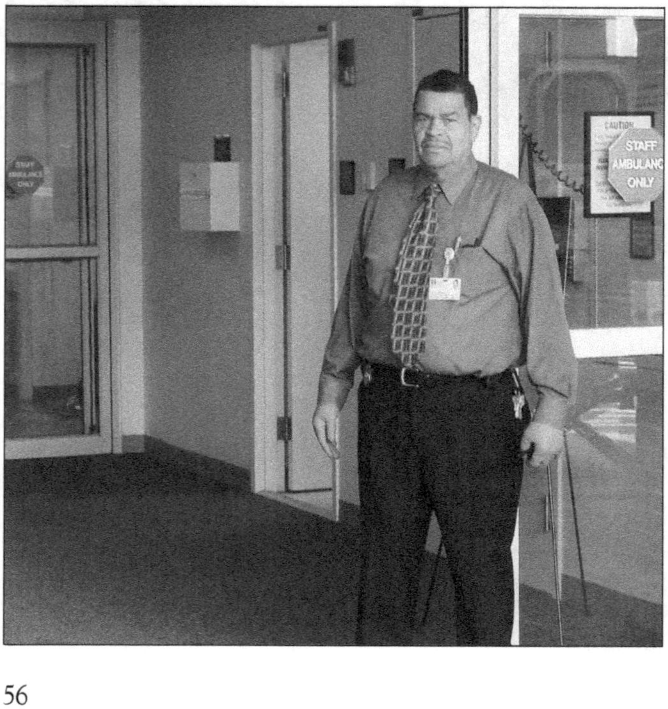

At the time of his death, Oliver "Ollie" Amado Jr. had been senior operations coordinator of public safety at South Shore Hospital for more than 19 years. Ollie embodied the culture and spirit of hospital employees, always cheerfully devoting extra effort to ensure that everyone was secure and well served, whether the former president of the United States or a homeless patient.

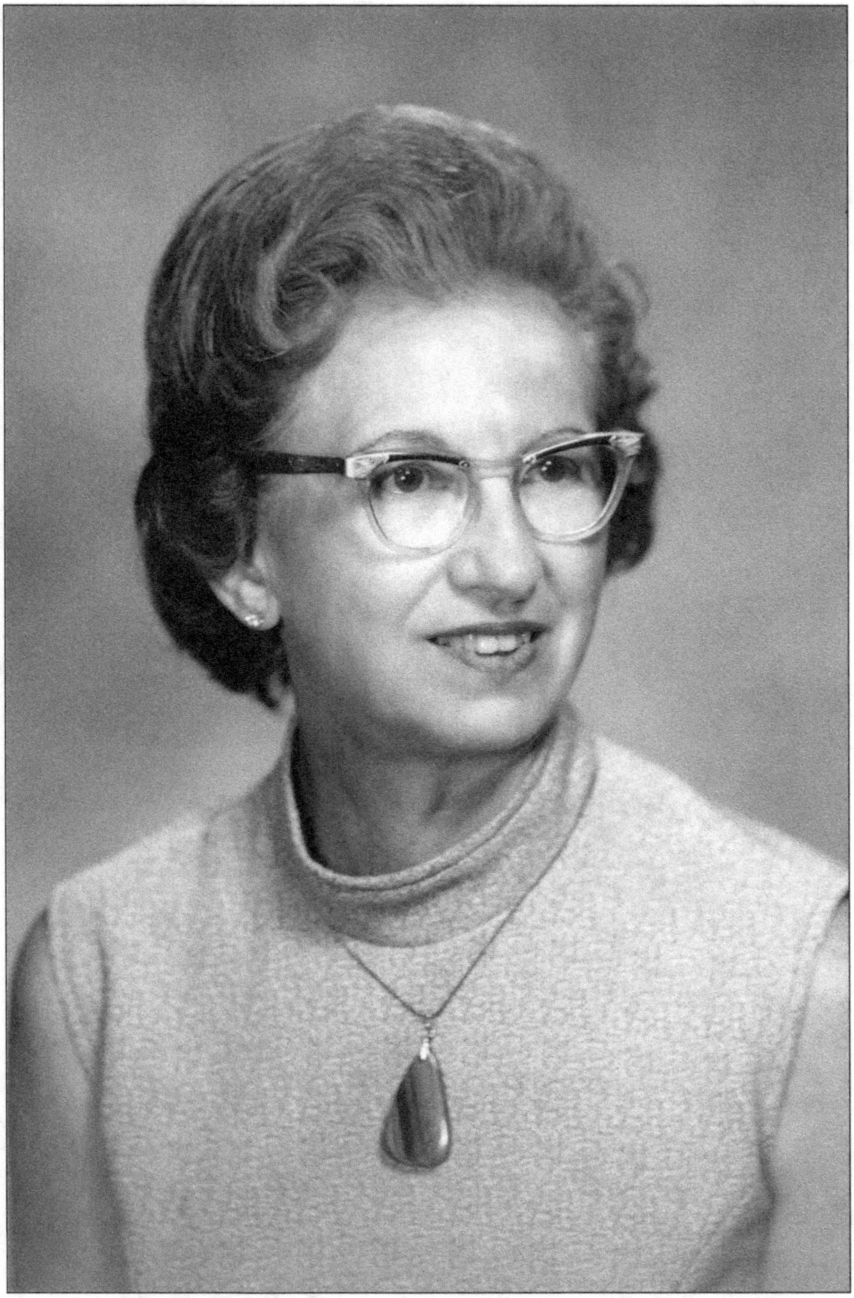

Mary Corbett was devoted to the hospital's mission. Her 44-year career began in 1944. As the office manager, she was responsible for signing all checks and kept accounts in a 12-column ledger. She was the first female president of the Hospital Financial Management Association's Massachusetts chapter. After retiring as comptroller, she amassed 3,000 hours as a hospital volunteer. She also contributed significant financial skills to the Friends of South Shore Hospital and volunteered in the Foundation, organizing the accounting for special donor funds. Known for her intelligence, common sense, and New England frugality, this longtime Weymouthian was steadfast and generous to the charity she loved, even after she died. She bequeathed over $1 million to the hospital. In gratitude for her generosity, the hospital named its popular dining room in her honor.

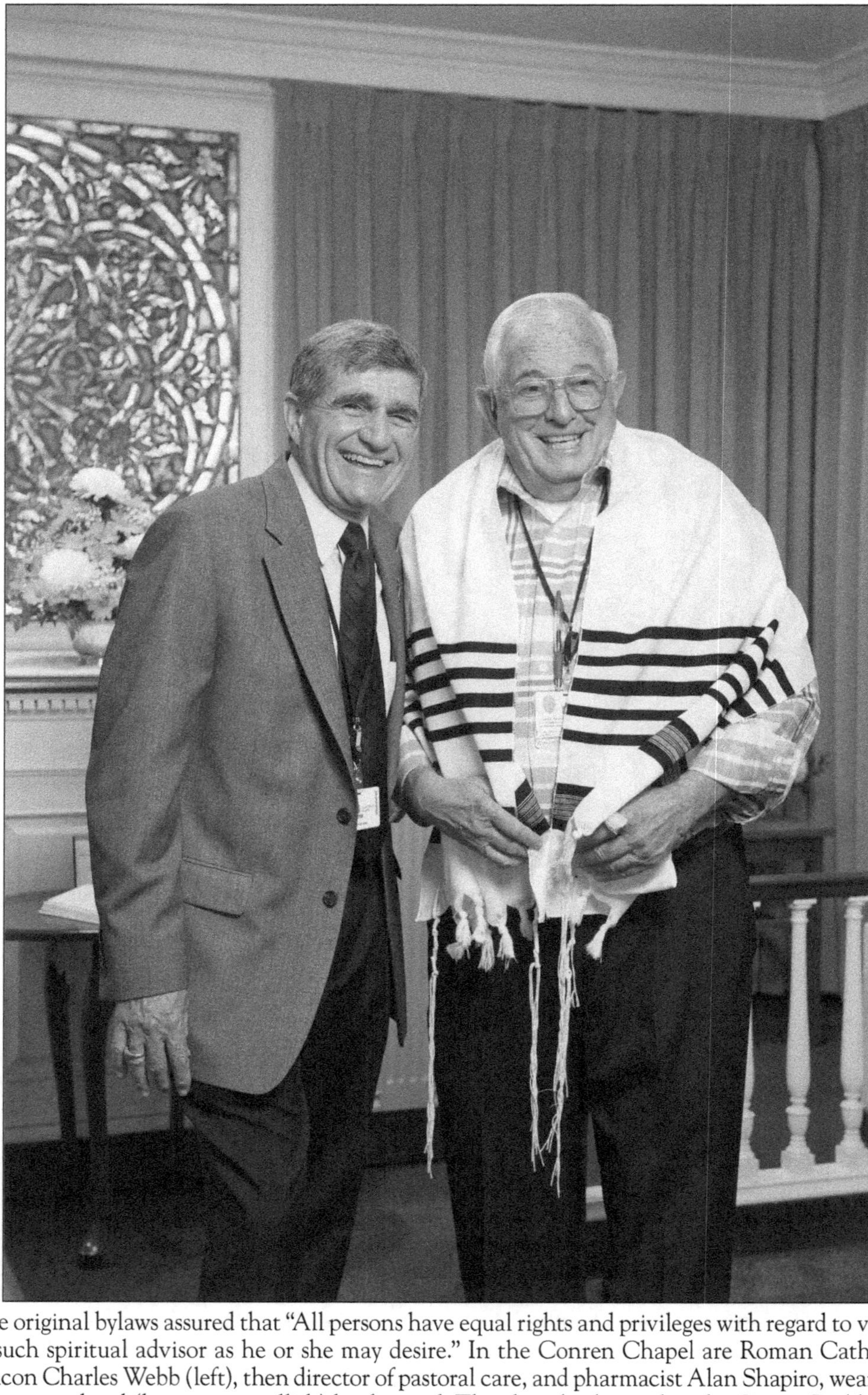

The original bylaws assured that "All persons have equal rights and privileges with regard to visits of such spiritual advisor as he or she may desire." In the Conren Chapel are Roman Catholic deacon Charles Webb (left), then director of pastoral care, and pharmacist Alan Shapiro, wearing the prayer shawl (known as a tallith) he donated. The chapel is located in the Center Building's former lobby.

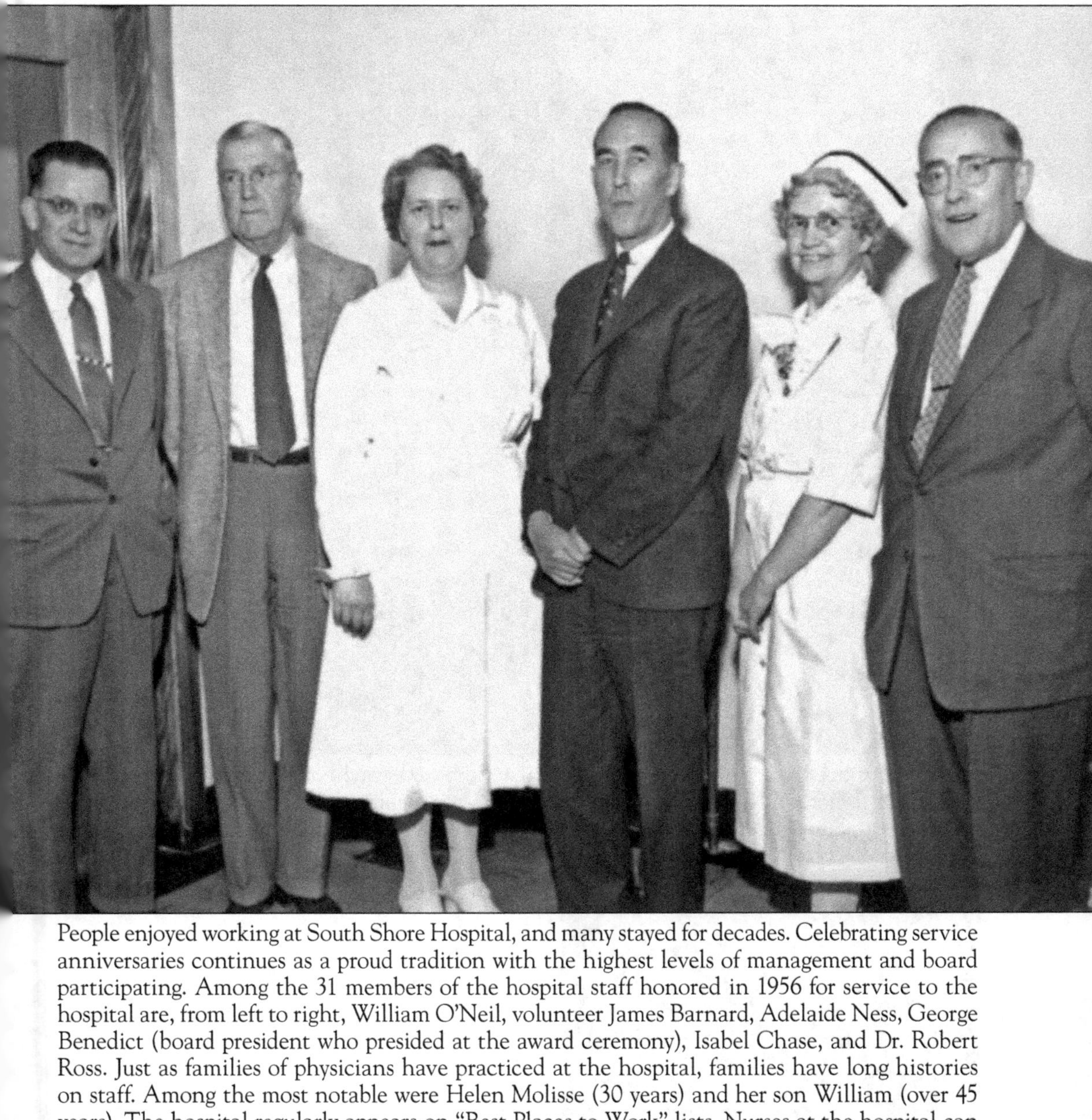

People enjoyed working at South Shore Hospital, and many stayed for decades. Celebrating service anniversaries continues as a proud tradition with the highest levels of management and board participating. Among the 31 members of the hospital staff honored in 1956 for service to the hospital are, from left to right, William O'Neil, volunteer James Barnard, Adelaide Ness, George Benedict (board president who presided at the award ceremony), Isabel Chase, and Dr. Robert Ross. Just as families of physicians have practiced at the hospital, families have long histories on staff. Among the most notable were Helen Molisse (30 years) and her son William (over 45 years). The hospital regularly appears on "Best Places to Work" lists. Nurses at the hospital can participate in professional education through Simmons College, for example. As part of its culture of caring, the hospital insists that colleagues are treated with respect.

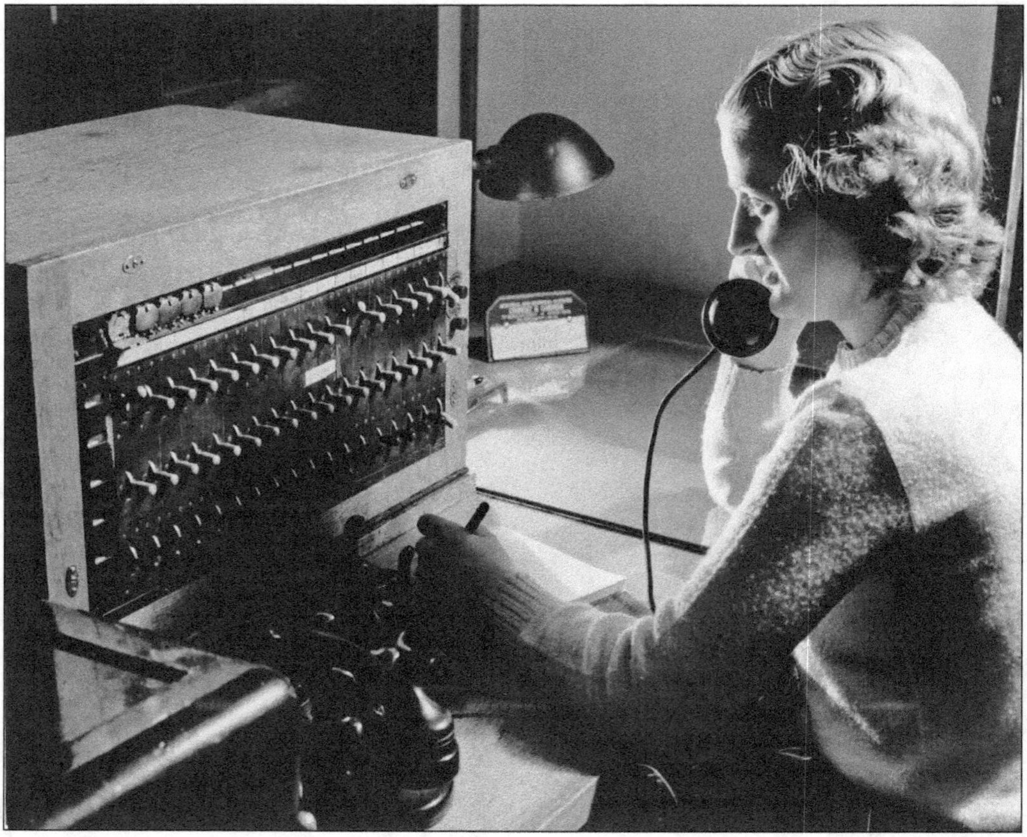

In this 1940 photograph, an operator uses a small wood-boxed switchboard to handle the hospital's calls. Next to her is a "French" phone, one of the first to combine a transmitter and receiver in the handset. Currently, the hospital's electronic switchboard handles hundreds of thousands of calls annually. (Photograph by William Rittase.)

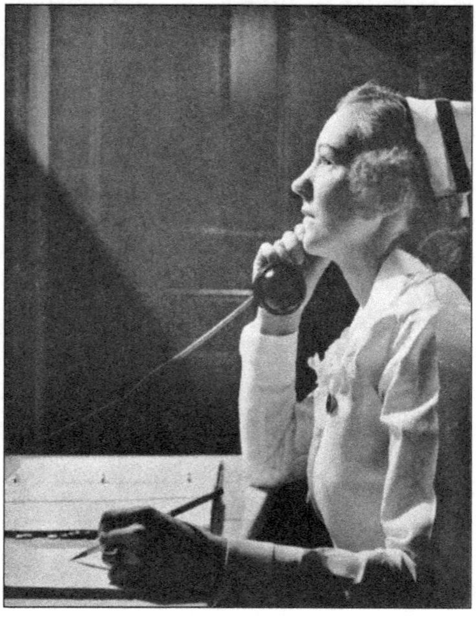

For this stylized 1940 photograph, a nurse wears a starched uniform, nursing pin, handkerchief, and cap with a black band, denoting the highest rank. Depending on the nursing school, students started with pink, blue, or other pastel ribbons. Rank could be revoked for poor behavior, like smoking in the hospital. Soon after World War II, caps were worn less frequently. Paper replaced starched fabric. As men entered nursing and feminism grew, caps disappeared.

Five

PATIENT CARE
"WITH EXPERTISE, COMPASSION, AND RESPECT"

Hospital president Arthur Perkins thus described how care was provided 50 years ago. The hospital exists to care for patients. Because this is the core activity, its quality is monitored closely. Independent accrediting organizations and government agencies ranked the hospital's medical staff, nurses, clinicians, services, and facilities as among the country's best. It was ranked higher than most hospitals in the country by the Joint Commission, the "gold standard" for measuring quality.

In those early days, patients had to travel by streetcar to Boston for care, especially from specialists. As South Shore Hospital proved its ability to treat more complex conditions, world-renowned Boston hospitals, including Children's Hospital Boston, sought clinical affiliations with South Shore. South Shore Hospital is the only community hospital licensed to provide Level III maternal and child care, including a neonatal intensive care unit. The hospital collaborated with Dana-Farber Cancer Institute and Brigham and Women's Hospital to provide the highest levels of cancer care closer to South Shore residents in a state-of-the-art center.

The hospital has earned the confidence of its patients and the people of the region. As reported in independent surveys, nine of ten patients and their families would recommend the hospital to a family member or friends.

Buildings have been constructed; equipment has become more sophisticated. What has not changed is what patients expect. They want to trust their hospital. They want to feel safe and be kept informed. Patients want to be cared for as individuals—not as a collection of symptoms—with "expertise, compassion and respect."

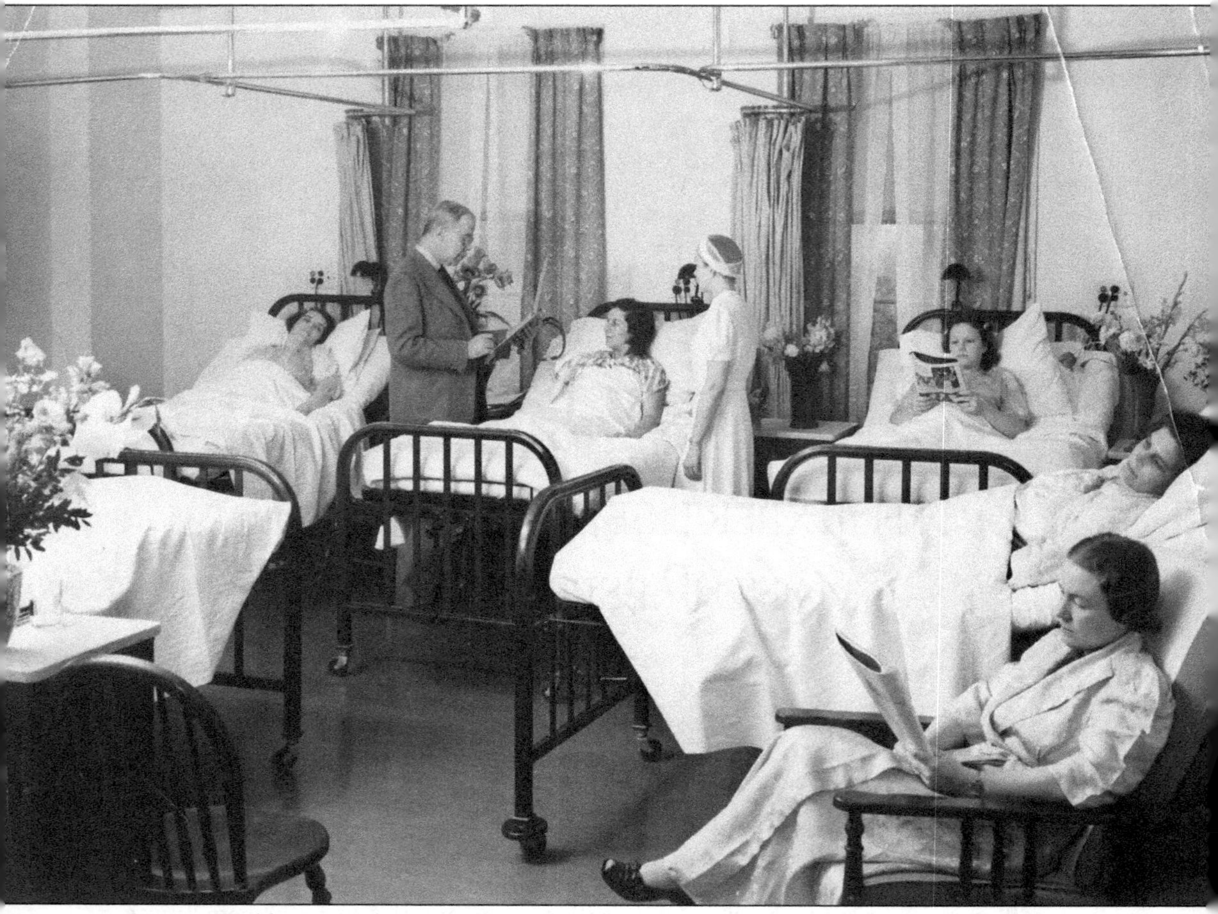

During World War II, the maternity ward that had opened a few years earlier was overcrowded. Privacy was minimal. Even after the mothers' stay was reduced from twelve to seven days, a radical step in 1942, every bed was filled. Births increased 22 percent from 1941 to 1943. With an occupancy rate of 90 percent or higher, there was no flexibility in moving the women elsewhere. More families moved into the area when the South Weymouth Naval Air Base opened. As soon as the Center Building opened in 1944, its maternity wards were filled. The baby boom exploded; 1,344 infants were born at the hospital in 1947, nearly double the births just six years previously. By 2011, annual births jumped to 3,800. The hospital's historic emphasis on quality earned it Massachusetts's highest possible licensure for maternity care, the same as academic medical centers.

Many hospital physicians and nurses enlisted during World War II, producing a shortage of nurses nationally and locally. Those working in hospitals devoted long hours and worked outside their job descriptions. It is remarkable that nurses took thousands of photographs of new mothers and their babies for fathers serving oversees, like that of Edith Morris (right) and her then unnamed child in May 1943. Even after the war, nurses celebrated babies' births, like that of Lorraine McSweeney and her daughter Lorraine (below) in 1962. Baby Lorraine was one of 2,132 births that year. Today, families, no matter how far-flung, can see their newborn's photographs on the hospital website.

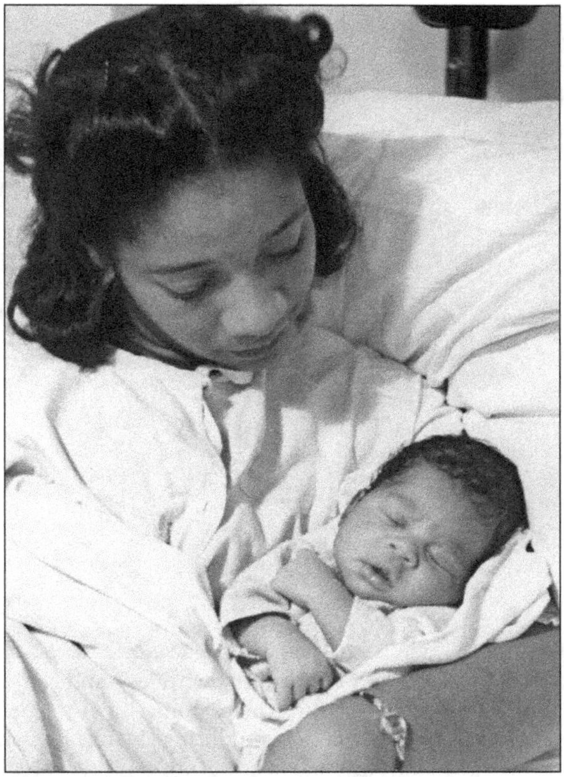

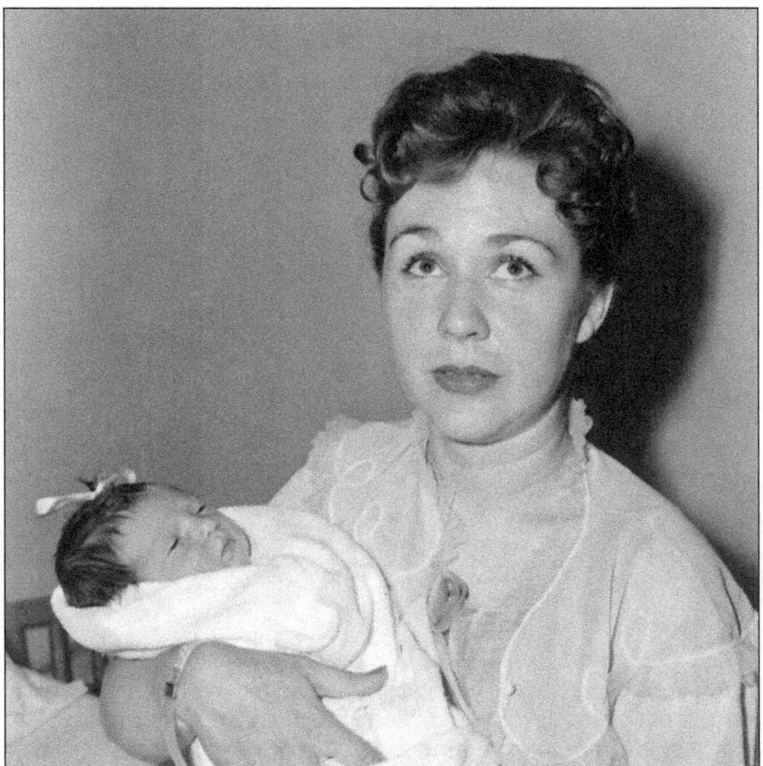

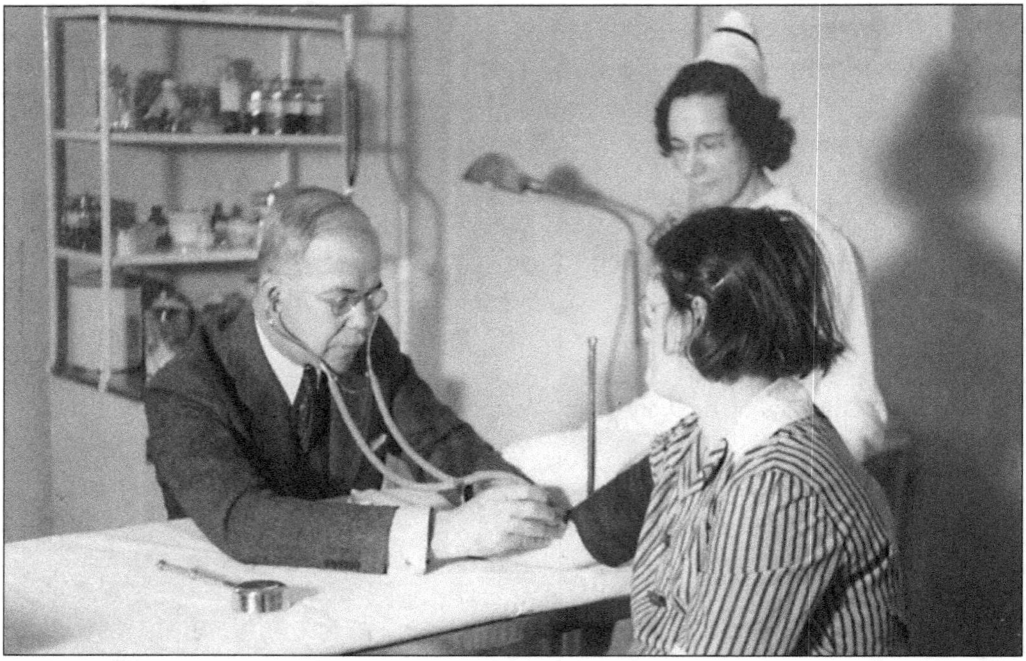

Chief of Obstetrics Dr. Wentworth Hoyt and nurse Katherine MacKay advise a mother-to-be at a 1936 prenatal clinic. At free clinics, physicians monitored the pregnancy and the mother's nutrition, especially important during the Depression and later wartime rationing. Penicillin was not yet available, and medications for high-risk pregnancies were limited.

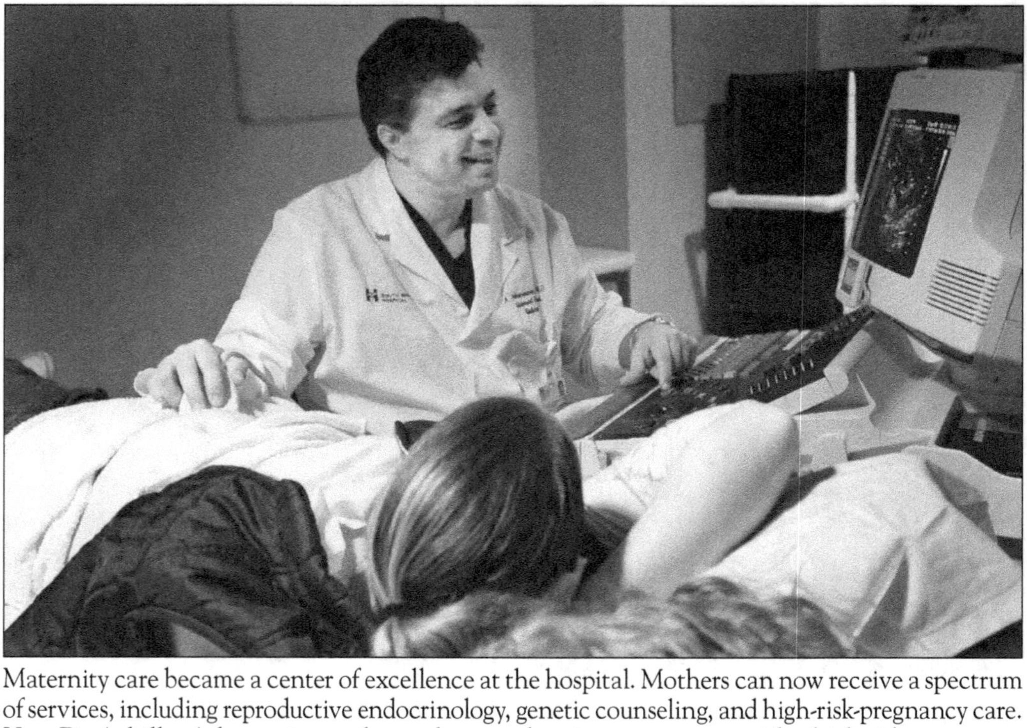

Maternity care became a center of excellence at the hospital. Mothers can now receive a spectrum of services, including reproductive endocrinology, genetic counseling, and high-risk-pregnancy care. Here Dr. Achilles Athanassiou performs ultrasound testing on a woman with a high-risk pregnancy. This extraordinarily expert level of care typically is available only at academic hospitals.

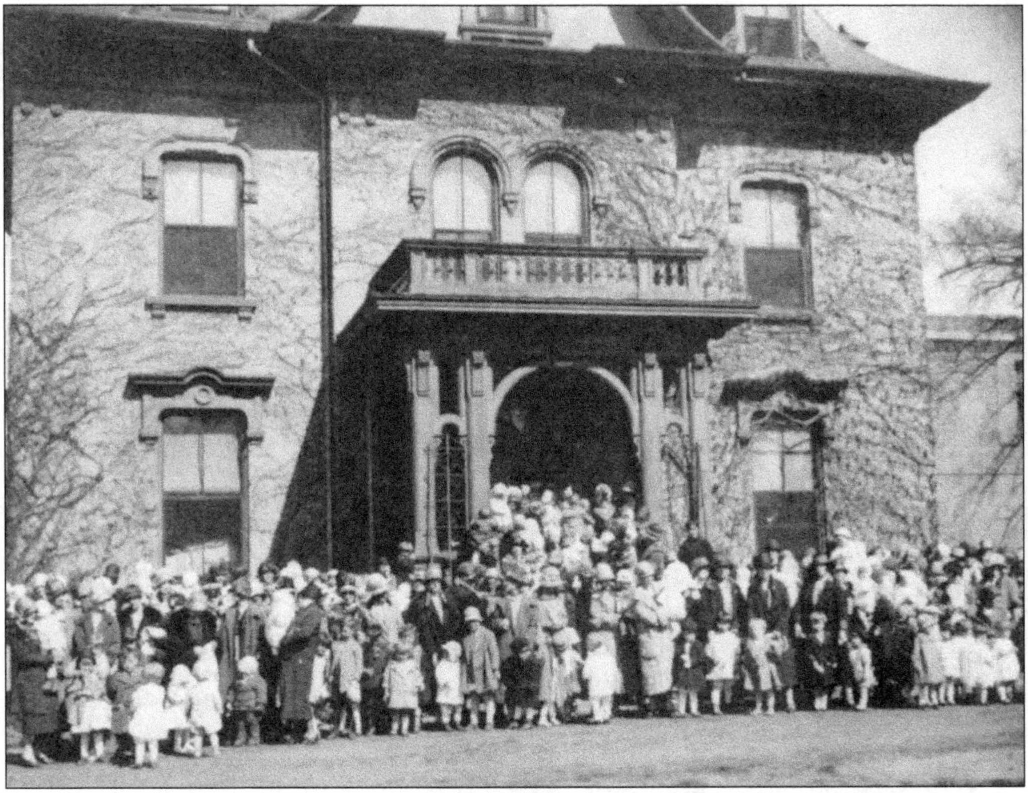

In 1945, hundreds of people born at the hospital gather for a reunion and pose for a photograph on the Reed Mansion's front steps. The first Weymouth Hospital baby, Joseph Weymouth DelMonaco, was born June 2, 1922. His middle name honored the hospital. Growing maternity services have propelled the hospital's expansion over the decades.

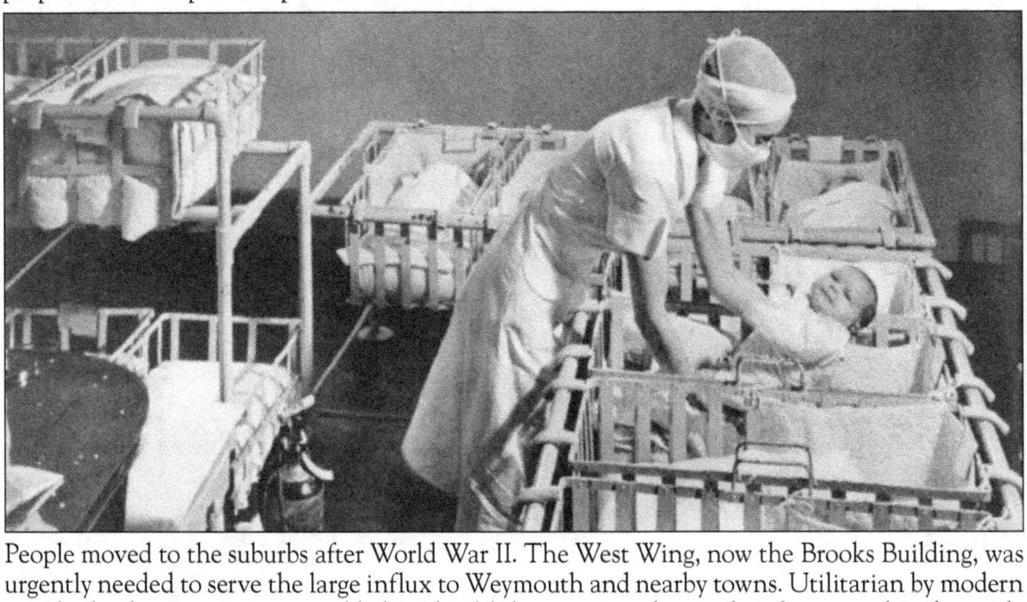

People moved to the suburbs after World War II. The West Wing, now the Brooks Building, was urgently needed to serve the large influx to Weymouth and nearby towns. Utilitarian by modern standards, the nursery improved babies' health by ensuring that each infant was placed in only one bassinet during its stay.

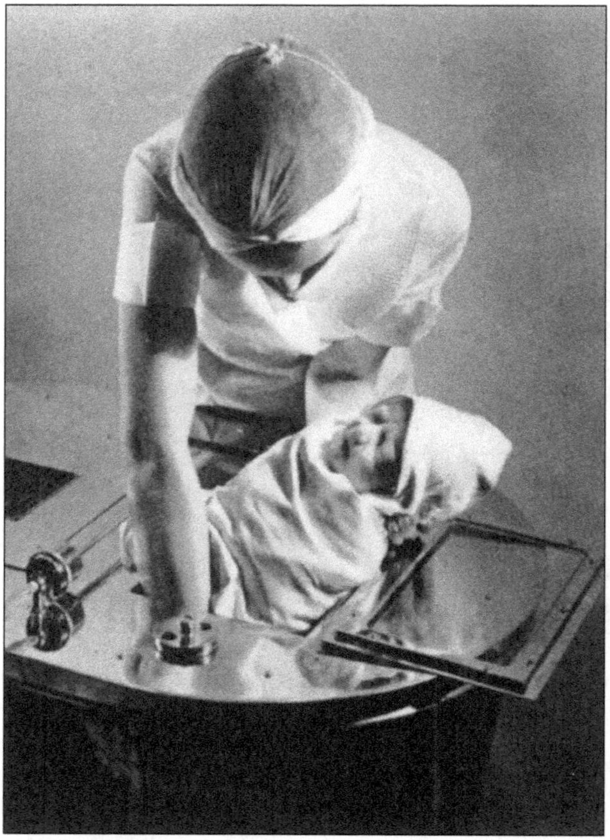

A nurse swaddles a baby before placing him in an incubator. Dr. Martin Couney invented incubators in the early 1900s. Physicians rejected them for 30 years until Couney created live baby-incubator displays at the New York World's Fair and in boardwalk storefronts in Coney Island and Atlantic City. The public watched as physicians and nurses cared for babies, who thrived. Below, nurses Phyllis Seppala (left) and Jeanne Hamala care for an infant in an isolette in the special care nursery. With its clear sides and top, and portals for nurses to touch the baby, this design was a huge improvement over the originals.

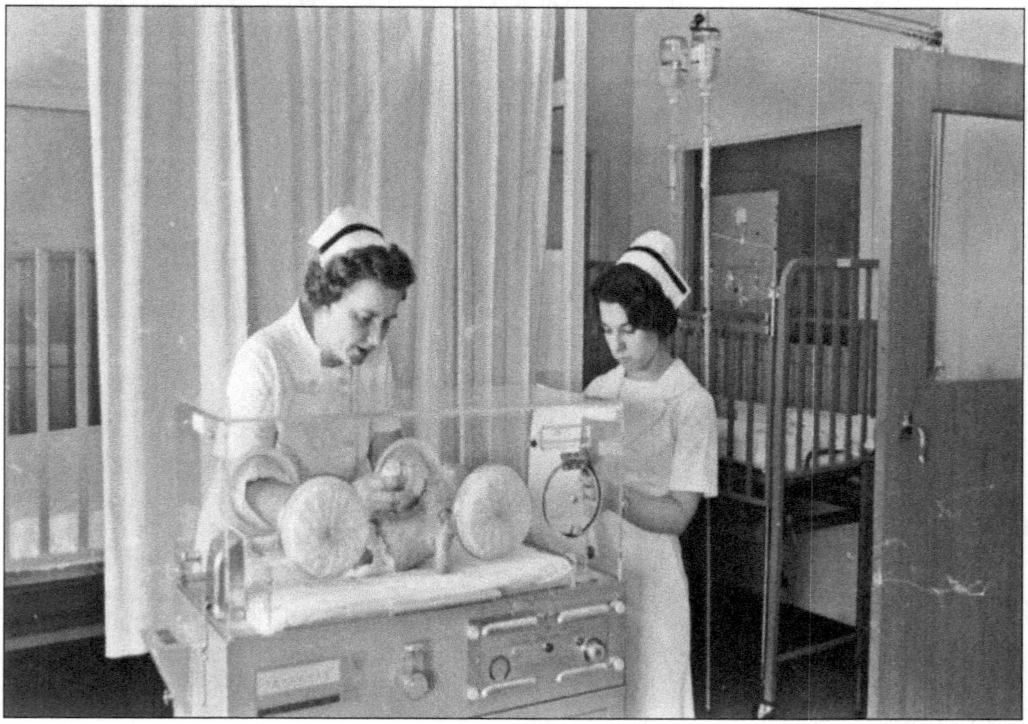

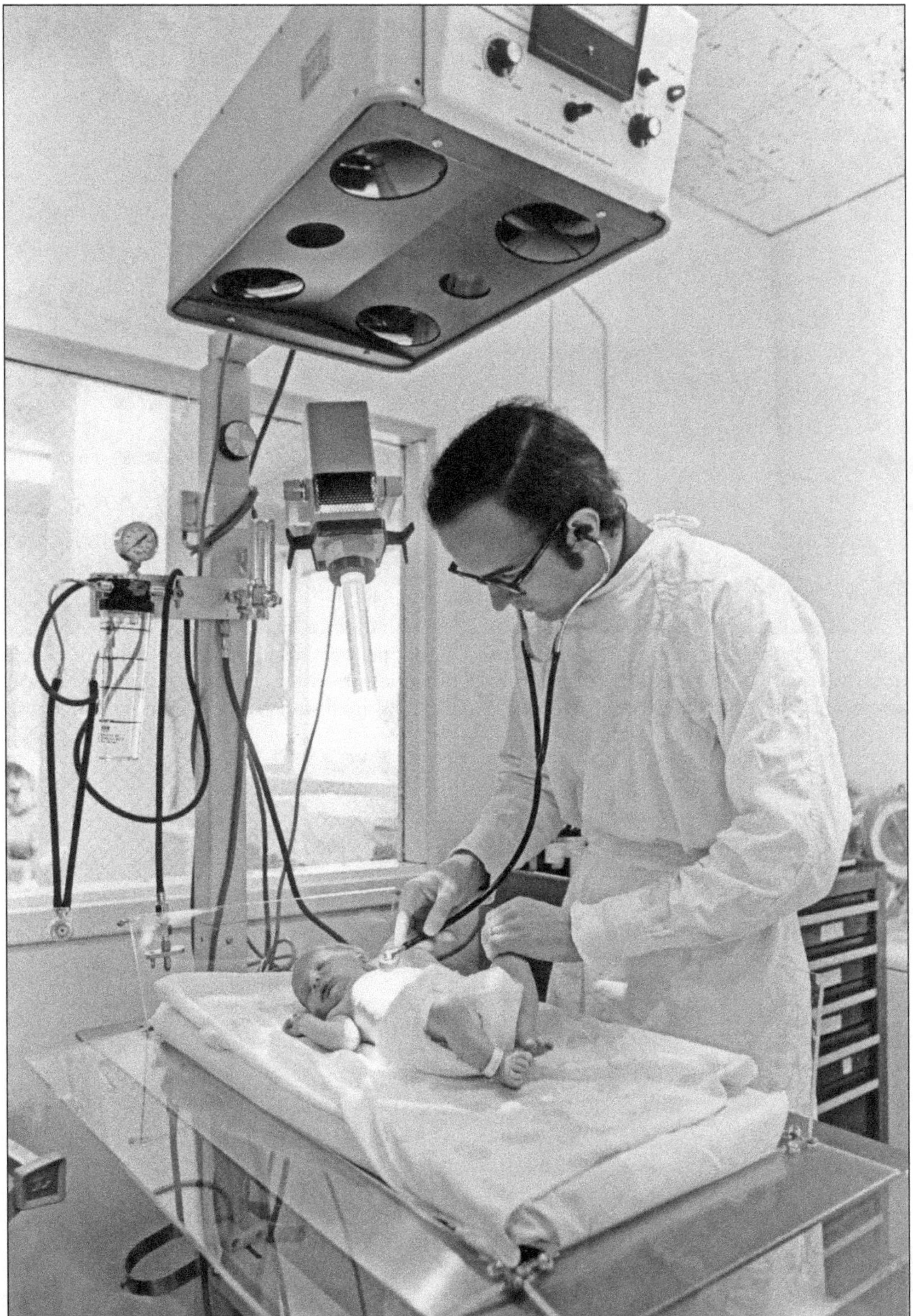

Dr. James Cox examines a high-risk newborn in the special care nursery, the first in the commonwealth at a community hospital. This nursery was designed for infants who need a level of care between the regular nursery and the Level III neonatal intensive care unit. With its critical and special nurseries, it is one of New England's largest and most comprehensive maternity centers.

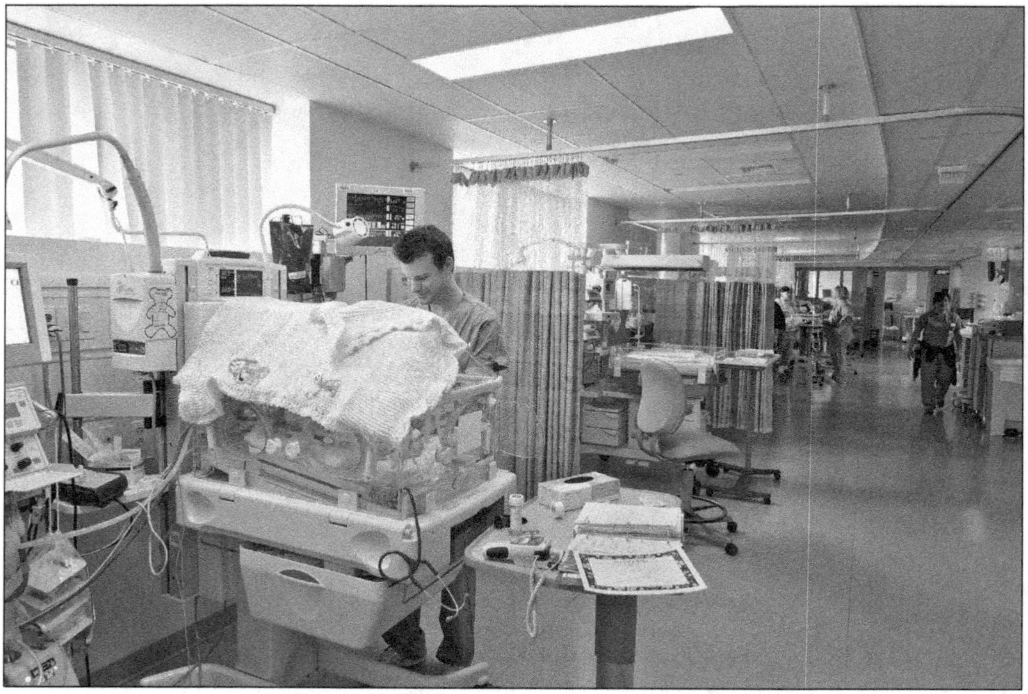

When the hospital was founded, a general practitioner performed surgeries and delivered babies. Similarly, there was no distinction in levels of nurseries, even for the most premature infants. Now, infants are more likely to survive, due to a highly skilled staff of 40 ob-gyns, certified nurse midwives, and 160 maternity nurses.

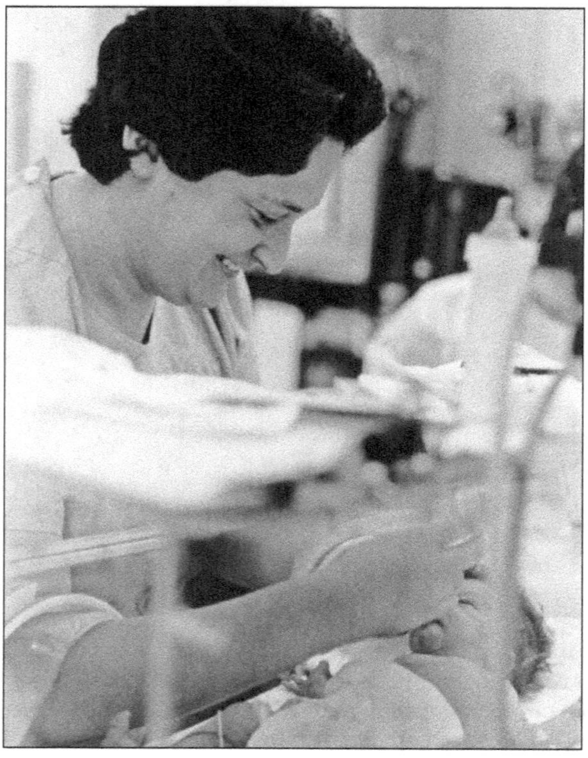

Nurse Marsha Cohen feeds a premature infant. Historically, most South Shore mothers chose to have their babies at the hospital. In 1923, in the hospital's first full year, 138 babies were born there, compared to 3,650 babies in 2010, including 95 sets of twins and triplets.

Nurse Pearl Hastay and an unidentified physician discharge a youngster in 1940. There were only five pediatric beds. Pediatric care was primarily provided in homes or physicians' offices. The new Center Building greatly increased the capacity for infants and children, especially due to Bryan Leonard's generosity. However, there was soon a waiting list for beds.

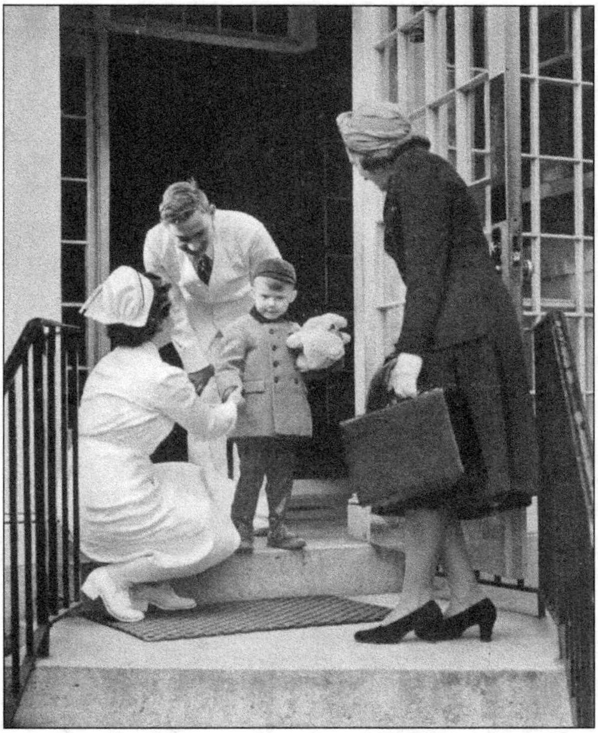

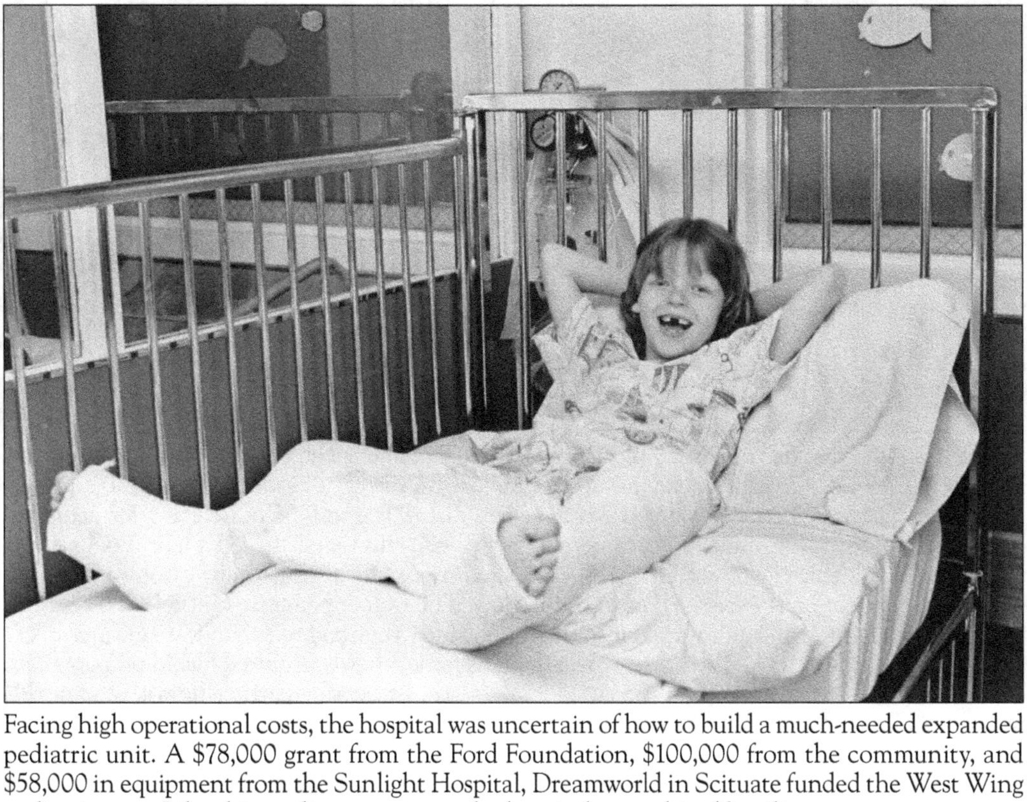

Facing high operational costs, the hospital was uncertain of how to build a much-needed expanded pediatric unit. A $78,000 grant from the Ford Foundation, $100,000 from the community, and $58,000 in equipment from the Sunlight Hospital, Dreamworld in Scituate funded the West Wing pediatric unit. Like this smiling youngster, the hospital proved itself resilient.

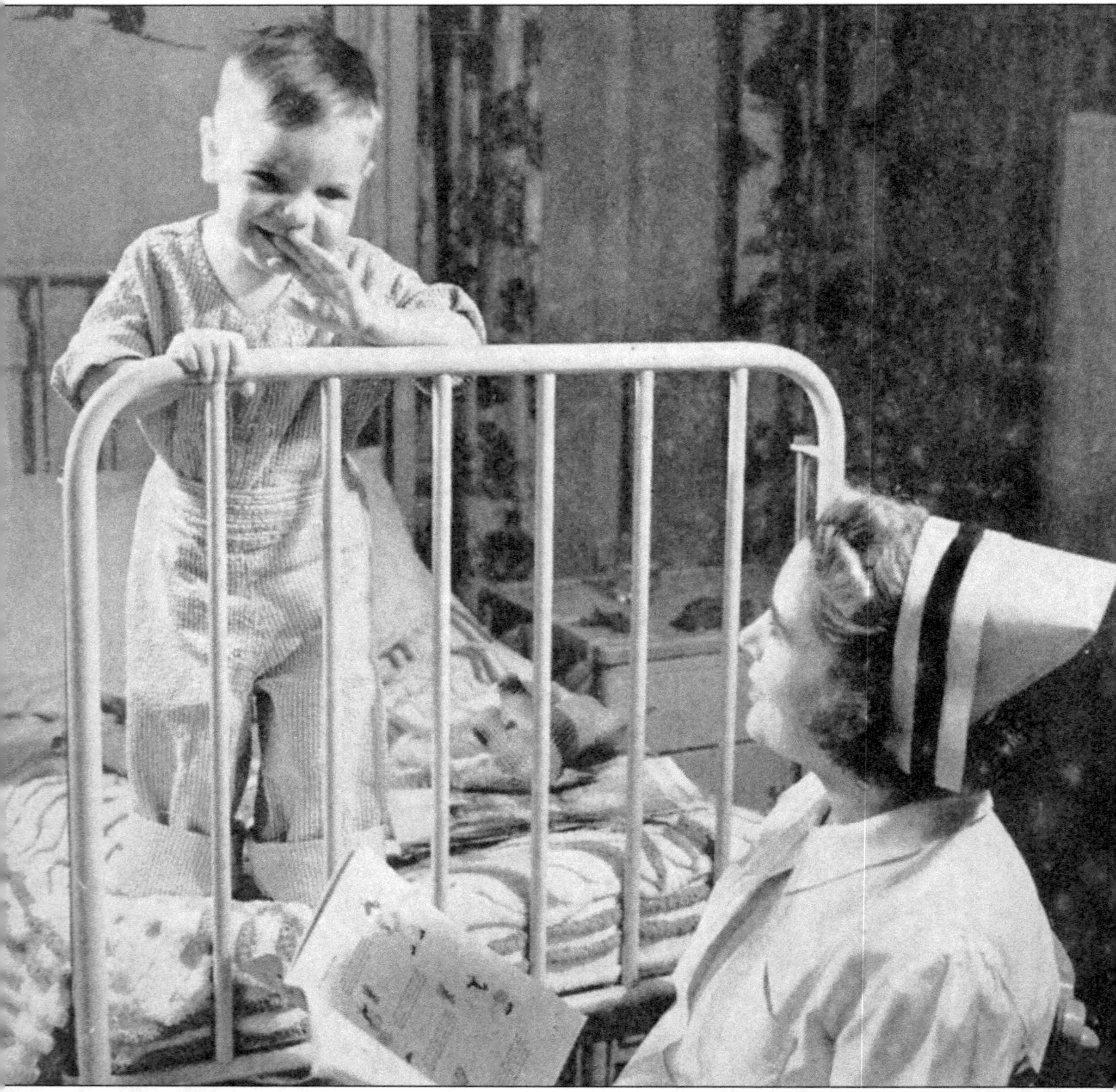

As the hospital expanded maternity services, it needed more pediatric beds. More infants survived birth, but some needed further care for congenital or chronic conditions. With 40,000 children in the region, Dr. Robert Ryan noted, "It has been disturbing to be required to refer pediatric cases to out-of-town hospitals . . . because of our own bed shortages." In 1957, a unit opened on the West Wing's third floor with 37 beds, compared to just 13 in the Administration Building where two corridor beds were filled most of the time. The former pediatric unit relieved pressure for beds by becoming an adult ward. Hospital leaders knew they had to expand. While architects were designing the pediatric unit, they created plans for the newly acquired Heald property east of the campus. Later, the hospital increased its pediatric services by partnering with the world-renowned Children's Hospital Boston.

An unidentified physician and nurse Nancy Lancaster treat a youngster with a broken leg. Below, nurse Patricia York adjusts a pillow for a youngster in traction. Children with emergencies were seen in the adult emergency department. However, children's medical issues often differ from those of adults. Parents in the region were pleased when the hospital launched a pediatric emergency service in conjunction with Children's Hospital Boston in 1998. The first of its kind in the region, it offered certified pediatric emergency care in partnership with Children's emergency physicians. Another benefit of this relationship was the introduction of neonatal intensive care and expanded inpatient and outpatient services for children with cardiac, gastrointestinal, and other complex conditions.

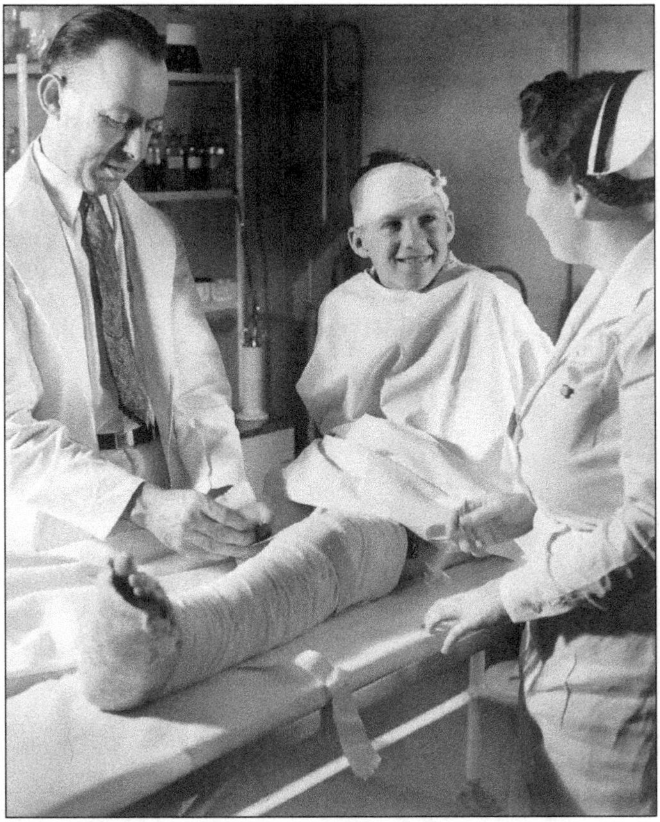

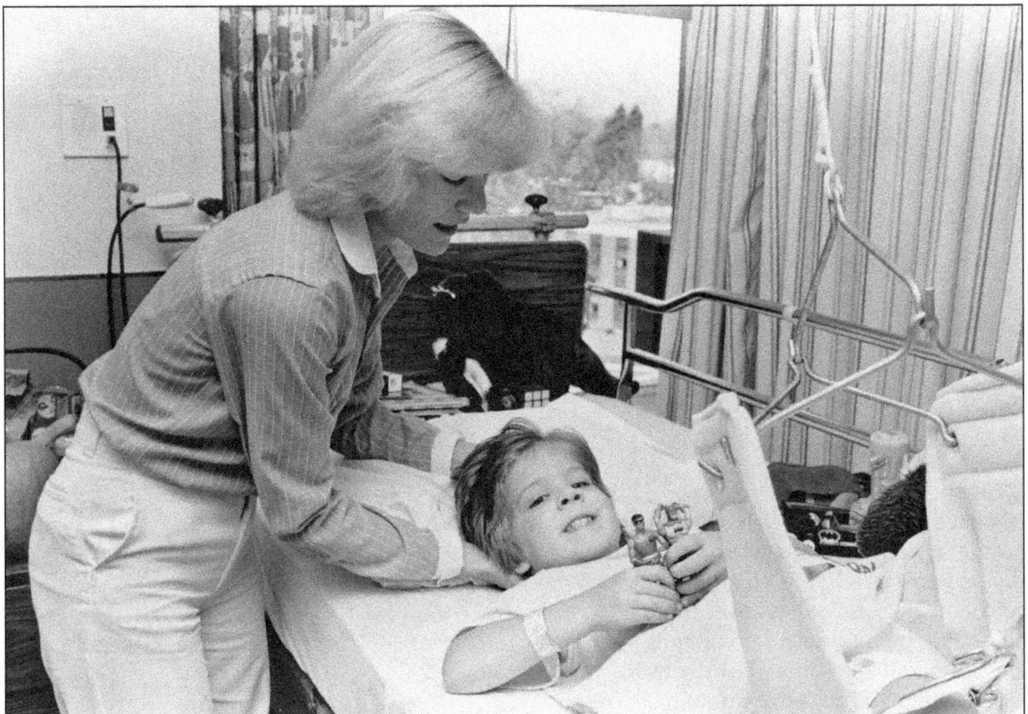

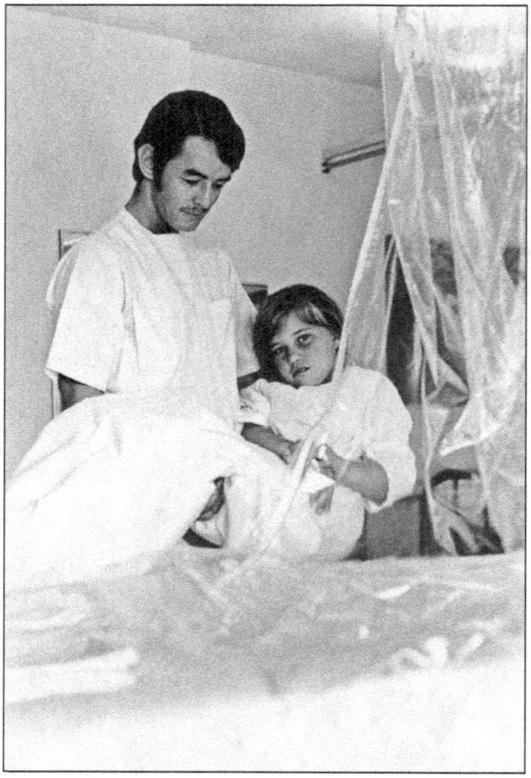

An orderly places a youngster with a respiratory condition into a transparent plastic oxygen tent. Tents were replaced with nasal cannulas (thin tubes with two small nozzles fitting into patients' nostrils) and face masks, all allowing more mobility and comfort. Now, at the hospital's wound care center, a hyperbaric chamber with 100 percent oxygen under greater-than-normal pressure helps wounds from radiation, trauma, and infections to heal faster.

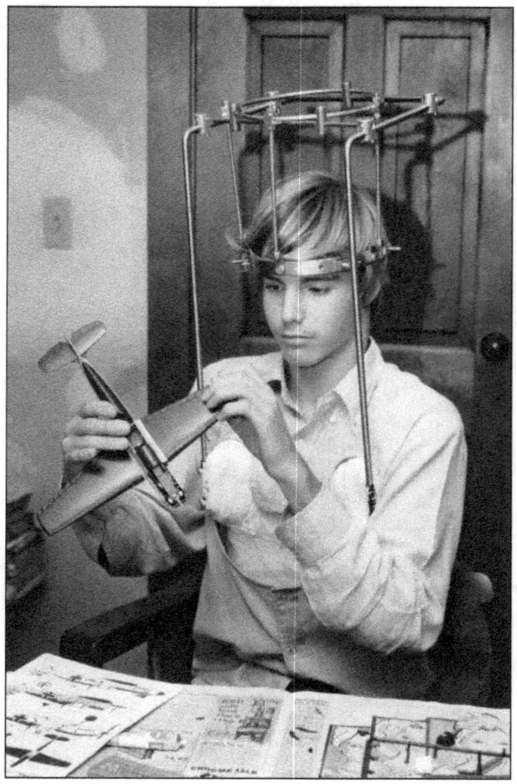

Michael Parker, of Norwell, would have been immobilized in traction when he fractured his cervical vertebra in an automobile accident. Because of advances in orthopedic care, like the halo cast, Parker built model airplanes and kept up with schoolwork. The hospital's physicians aim to heal and restore patients to their previous lifestyles.

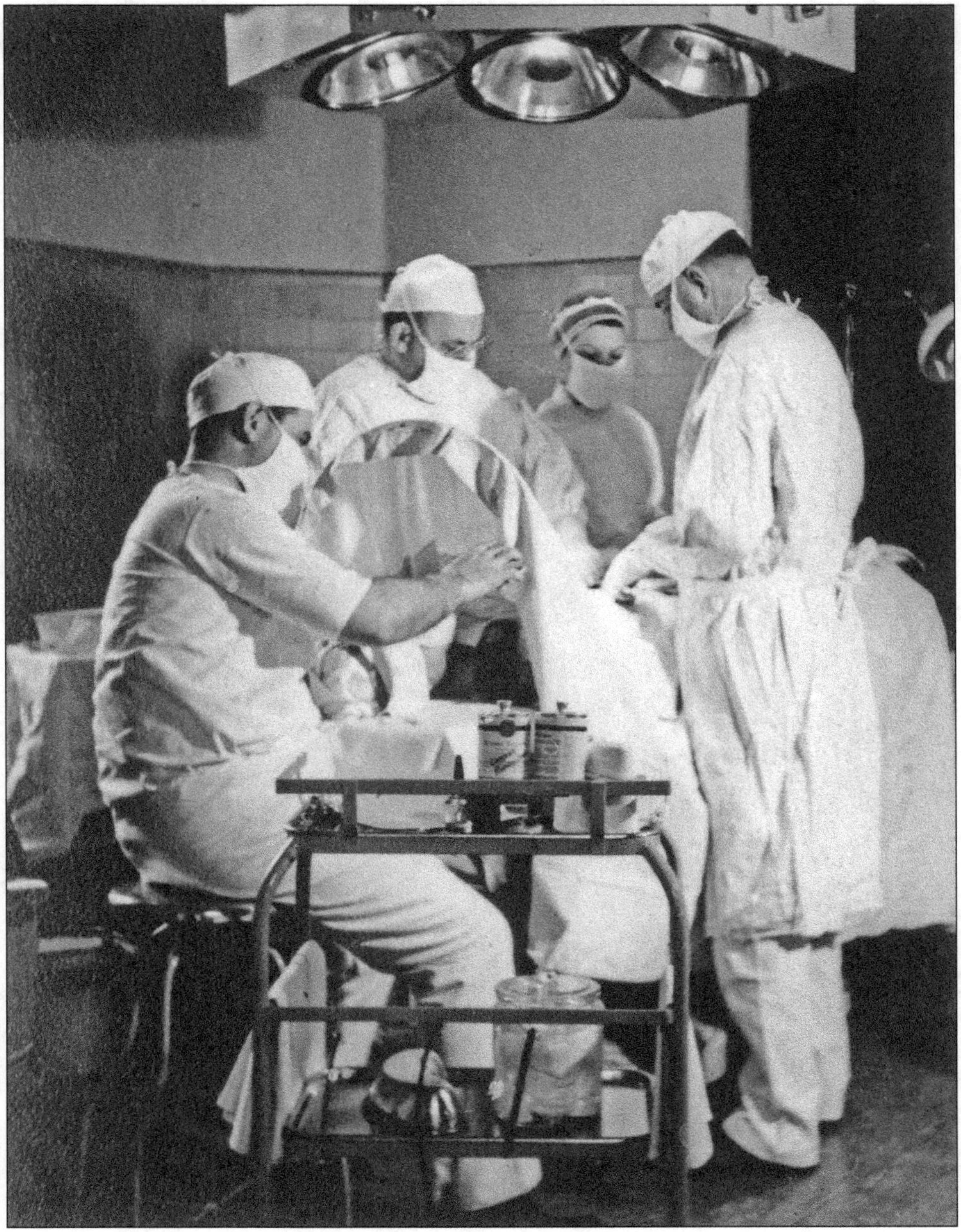

In 1940, an anesthesiologist (left) monitors a patient as two surgeons prepare to operate. A rolling cart holds containers of anesthesia and a glass jar of cloths in what was then considered a modern operating room. Through World War II, there was a long waiting list for surgeries. An explosion at the Old Colony Gas Company injured 18 people, reinforcing the need to expand. Wartime brought a large increase in other industrial accidents as hundreds of newly hired employees worked with munitions and heavy equipment. Nearby were the Hingham Ammunition Depot (supplying the entire North Atlantic theater of war), the National Fireworks Company in Hanover, the Navy's Fore River Shipyard in Quincy, and the South Weymouth Naval Air Station for Atlantic patrol dirigibles and antisubmarine warfare. A large migration caused over 475 houses, mostly single-family units, to be built in Weymouth in 18 months. The hospital had to expand again. (Photography by William Rittase.)

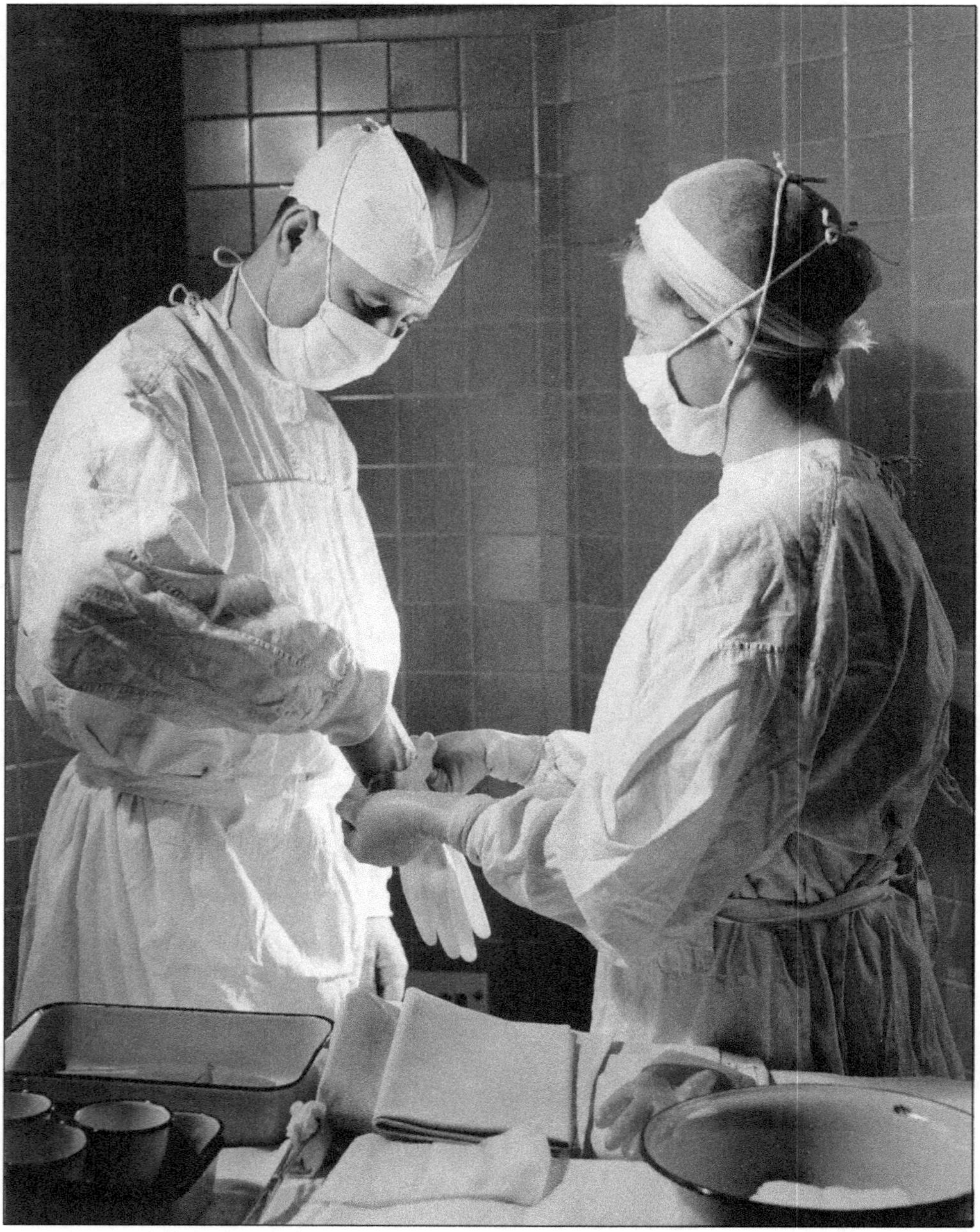

A paper-gowned physician and nurse prepare for surgery in the 1950s. A decade later, the hospital established the first day-surgery program at a community hospital in Greater Boston. Some 50 years later, surgeons use tiny cameras, miniature microscopes, fiber optics, voice-activated technology, robots, and high-definition monitors, along with traditional scalpels and sutures. The hospital surgical team is the region's largest, with 100 board-certified surgeons performing about 14,000 surgeries each year. From a single operating room on the second floor of the Reed Mansion, the hospital now has 14 operating suites in the Dr. James A. and Mary Lynd Dolphin Surgical Center. Day surgery is also done at the Center for Orthopedics, Spine, and Sports Medicine in Hingham. South Shore Hospital was named a Blue Distinction Center for Knee and Hip Replacement by Blue Cross Blue Shield for its quality of care and patient results in knee and hip replacement. (Photography by William Rittase.)

Pediatric emergencies can be frightening to the child and parents. Emergency medicine for children is different from adult care, requiring specifically trained physicians and different equipment. From a small accident room in the 1930s, the pediatric emergency department grew to the largest in the region, open 24 hours a day with thousands of visits a year.

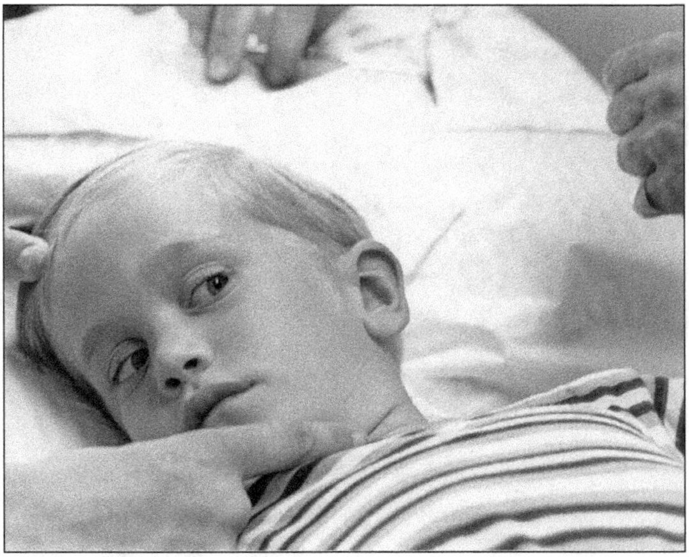

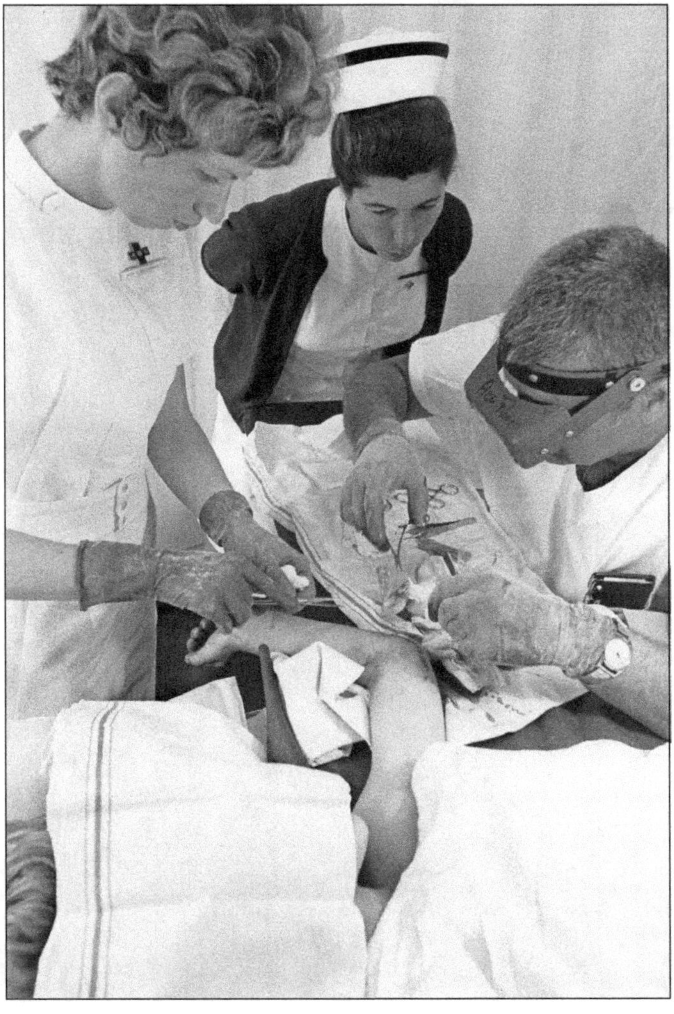

Nurses Georgia Buchanan (left) and Leslie Allen assist Dr. Matthew Jansics as he repairs a patient's elbow. With plastic surgeons, cardiologists, neurologists, and other board-certified physicians available, more complex and specialized procedures can be performed within the emergency department. It is one of the busiest emergency departments in the commonwealth with more than 85,000 visits annually.

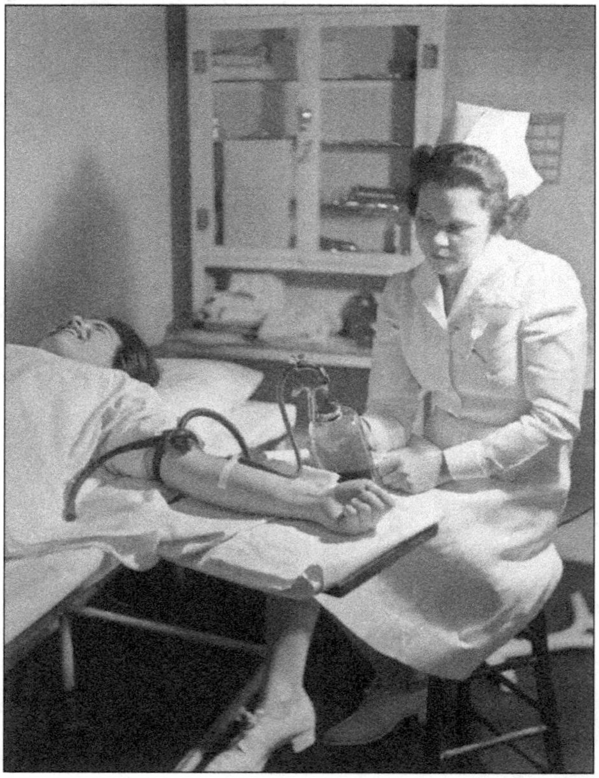

With nearly 2,000 surgeries and 1,344 births in 1947, the hospital plasma bank was busy. To augment staff, which included nurse Marie Conroy (shown here), the hospital hired Navy personnel to staff Wednesday and Saturday donor days. The hospital also provided blood for surgical patients at Norfolk County Hospital. Later, it offered the first on-site autologous blood program in the northeast with the Red Cross.

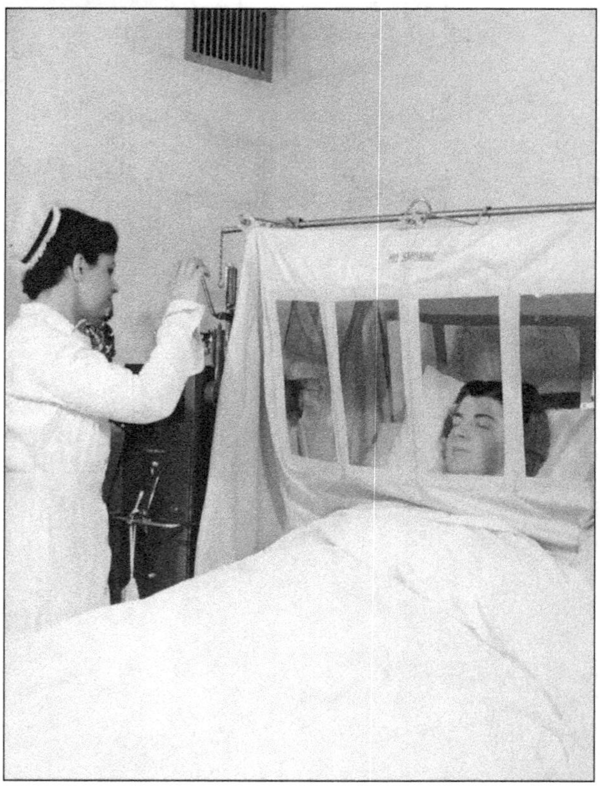

In 1939, nurse Marie Monaghan checks the oxygen flowing into a patient's tent. Intensive (critical) care became highly complex. The hospital's physicians are board-certified in intensive care and the nurses have special credentials. The hospital has the largest critical care units in the region and cares for more than 2,000 patients annually.

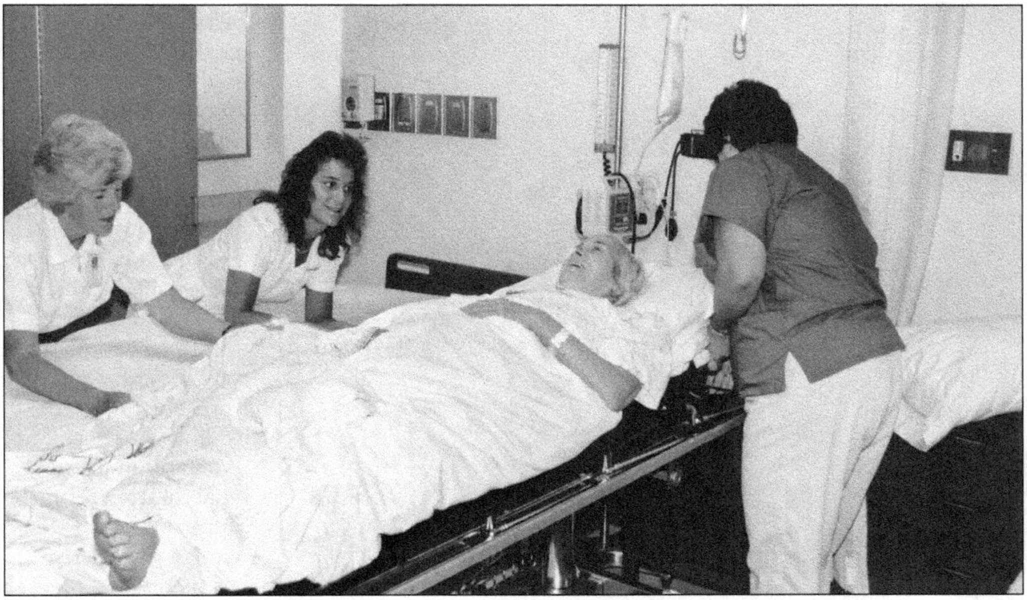

Nurse Nancy Shultz (left) and two unidentified nurses move the first patient into the 60-bed Emerson Building in 1989. The Emerson Building had three times as many beds as the original hospital and was named in honor of the founding physician, Dr. George Emerson. Ground was broken for a 60-bed addition in 2011.

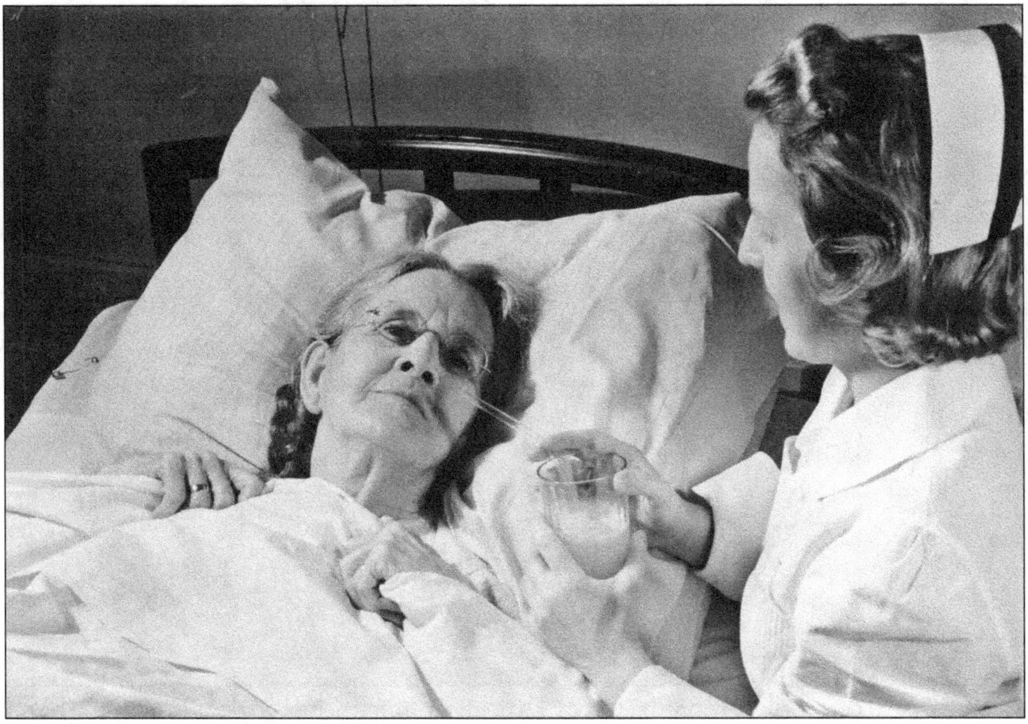

A nurse assists a patient in 1940. Nurses still provide friendly expert care, albeit without the starched uniform and cap. Although nursing assistants help with some activities, South Shore Hospital is one of a few in Massachusetts where only registered nurses provide bedside care. This standard, among others, earned the nursing staff the coveted national Magnet status.

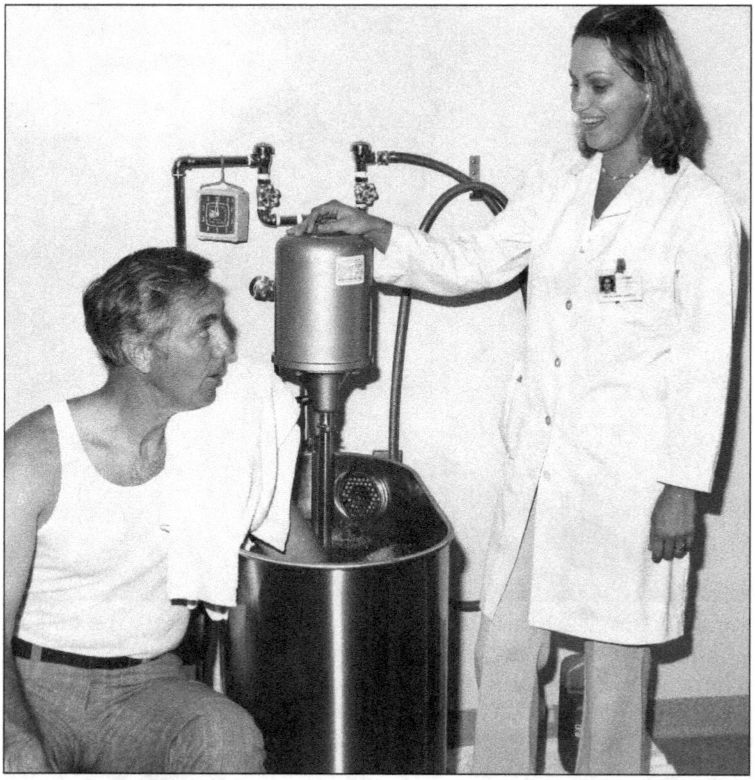

Before electronic monitoring, therapists used tried-and-true procedures like hydrotherapy. Notice the wind-up timer attached to the pipe. Both patient and therapist are unidentified. During World War II when untrained people were hired for factory work, the hospital expanded its accident room and industrial rehabilitation services. Since then, the number of patients has increased, often dramatically.

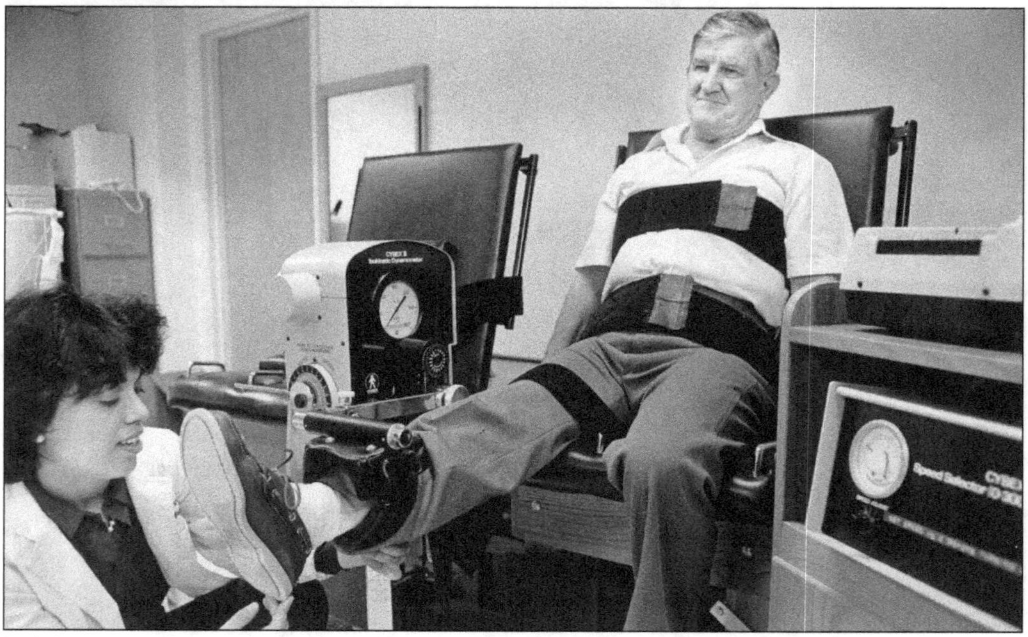

Ralph Farrar receives therapy on the Cybex Dynometer from therapist Priscilla Scoccia. (As a Hospital volunteer, Farrar accumulated the most hours ever.) Although an improvement over the previous rehabilitation facilities, space was tight. Equipment became more specialized and required an increasing investment. The 2011 opening of the Center for Orthopedic, Spine, and Sports Medicine in Hingham consolidated advanced care into one setting.

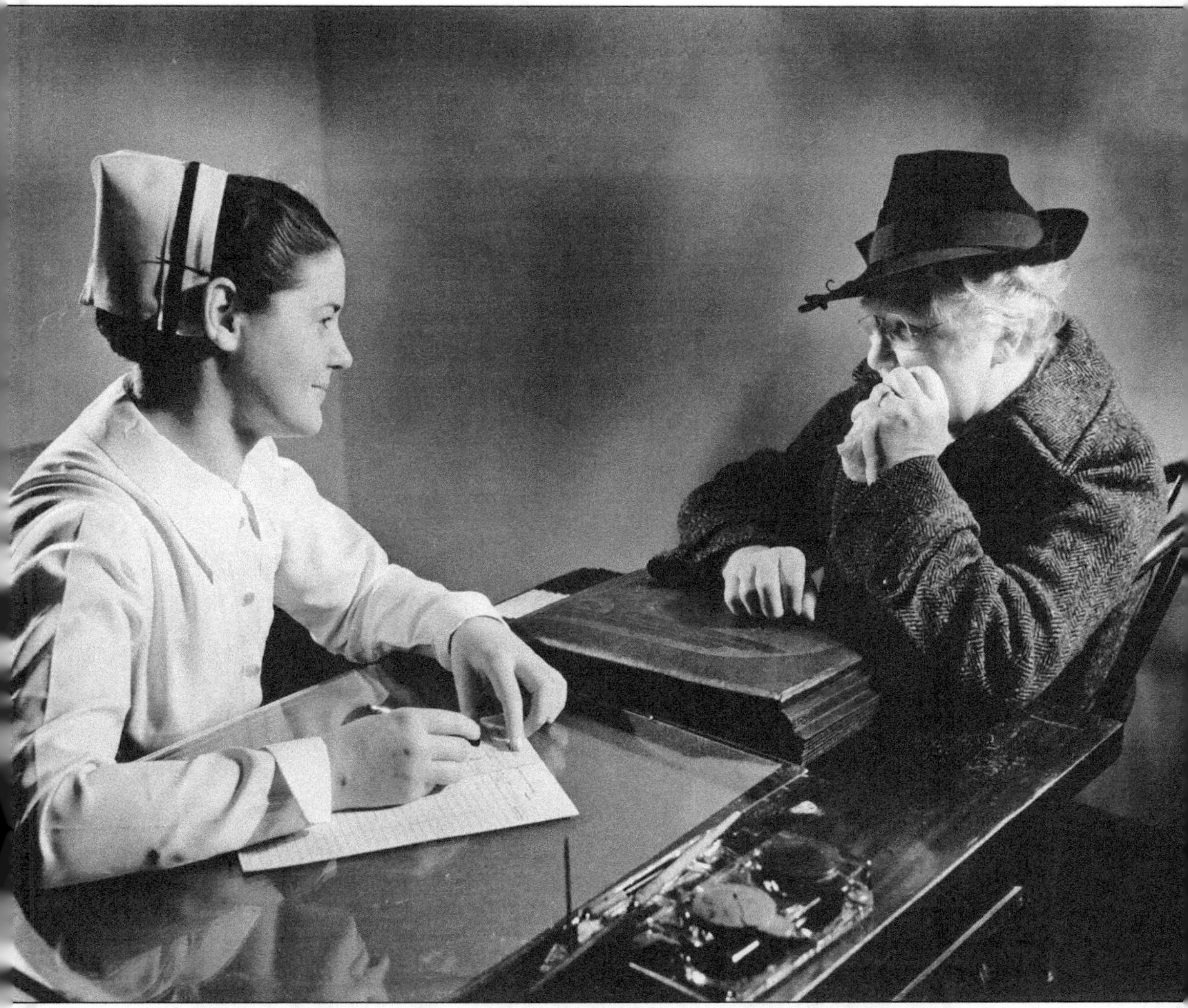

As stated in its original bylaws, the hospital provided care regardless of a patient's ability to pay. At times, this produced large deficits made up by donations from trustees and other generous donors. To make care more affordable and to level spikes in payments, the hospital became the first New England hospital to institute a radical new idea: group hospitalization insurance. Known as the Weymouth Hospital Service Plan, its rates were $12 per person per year, $19 per couple, and $7 each for additional family members. A precursor to Blue Cross Blue Shield, the plan entitled its 1,300 enrollees to three weeks of free care, including surgery and maternity. By 2010, the hospital provided almost $40 million in free care and other community benefits annually. This photograph was taken to raise funds in 1940 to build the West Wing (now the Brooks Building). (Photograph by William Rittase.)

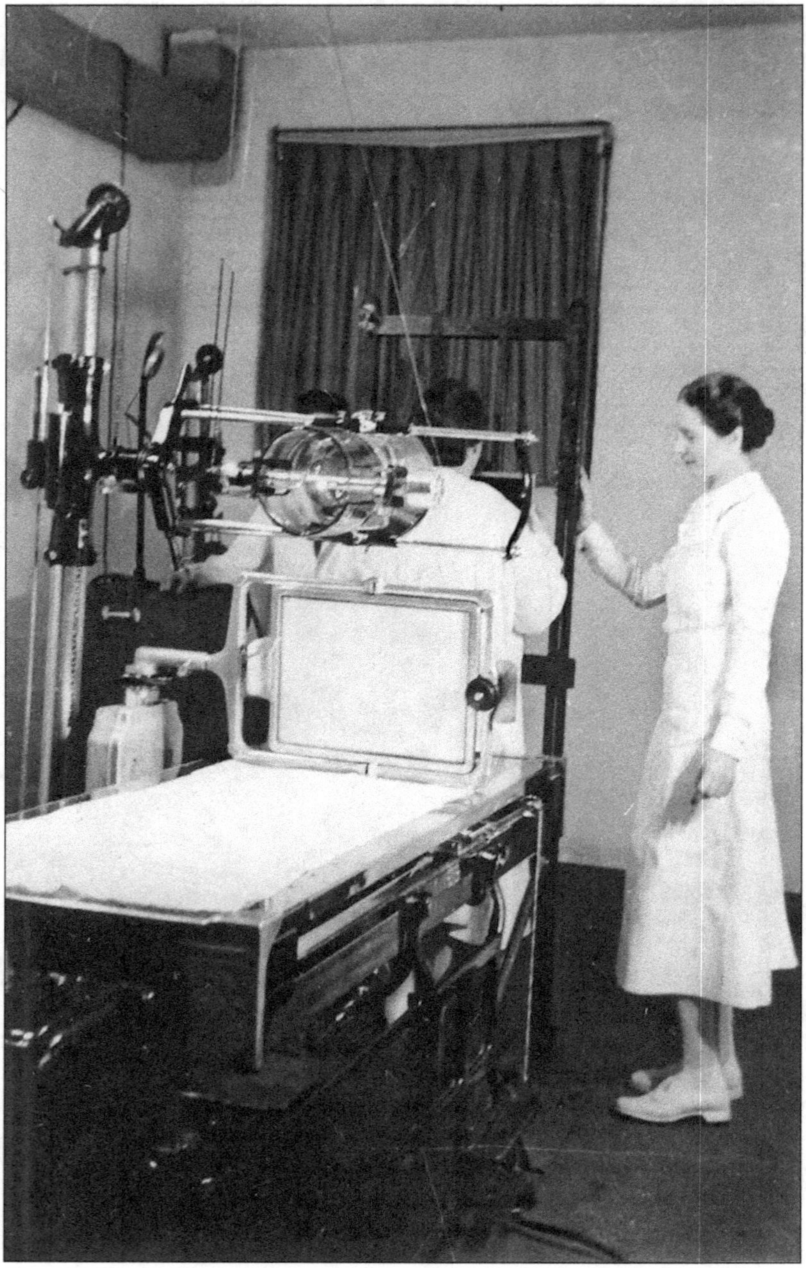

The hospital consistently invested in advanced and expensive scanners. Virtually every addition included expanded radiology: from the refitted Reed Mansion in 1922 to the new orthopedic center that opened in 2011. The $7,500 Picker X-ray machine was a major improvement over the original 1930s equipment that had reached the end of its usefulness, according to Roentgenologist Folke Wicklund. (Radiologists were known then as roentgenologists in honor of Wilhelm Conrad Röntgen who discovered X-rays.) With the new model, the patient stood tightly against a special, heavy screening stand, suitable for intensive examinations of the chest. The machines also had an automatic timer, although nurses also used push-button timers. X-ray screenings cost $10 each. In the 1930s and 1940s, X-rays were thought to be a panacea. A 1939 issue of *Mechanix Illustrated* effused, "The X-ray is more than a tool of the surgeon. It is a force in the change of civilization."

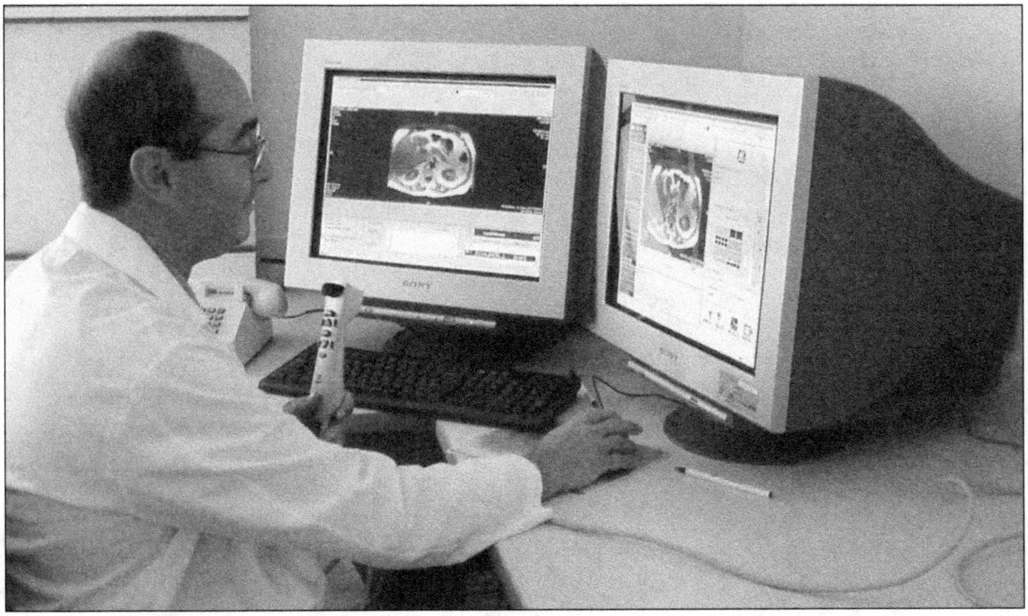

Dr. James Bezreh reviews a scan in the radiology suites in the Laban Pratt Building, which opened in the 1970s, then the most modern in the region. More precise diagnosis is possible with computerized tomography (CT), magnetic resonance imaging (MRI), and positron emission tomography (PET) scanners, all now available for examining bone, soft tissue, and tumors.

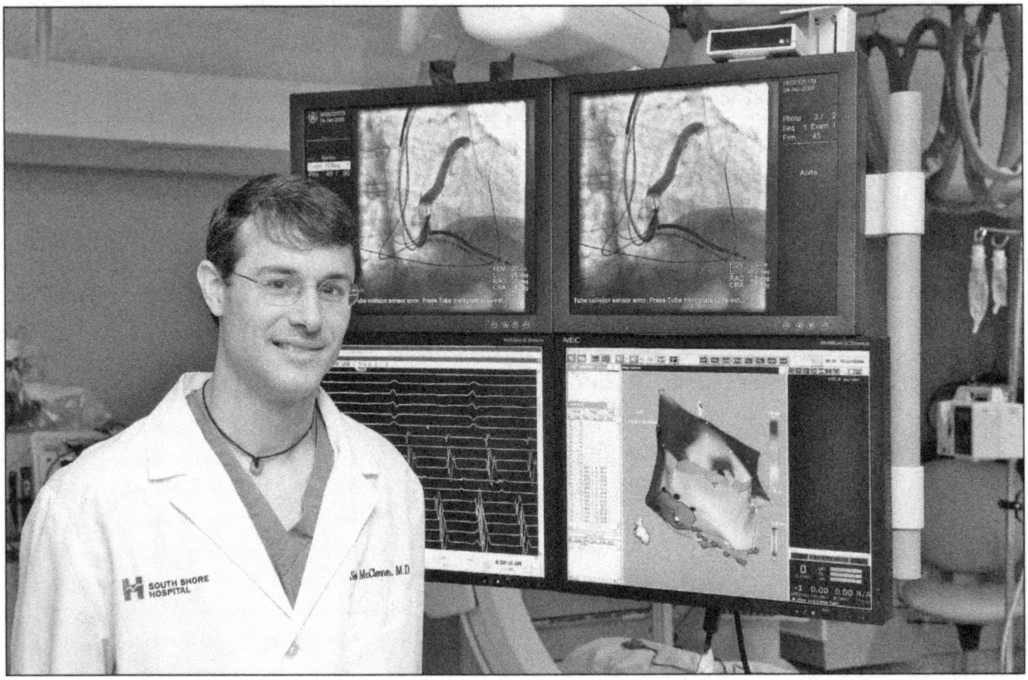

With the latest iteration of viewing diagnostic scans, South Shore Hospital cardiologists, like Dr. Seth McClennen, can view the heart three dimensionally and rotate the image. South Shore Hospital was one of the commonwealth's first community-based hospitals performing both emergency and elective angioplasty. Almost 3,000 of these life-saving procedures are performed a year, more than at any other community hospital in Massachusetts.

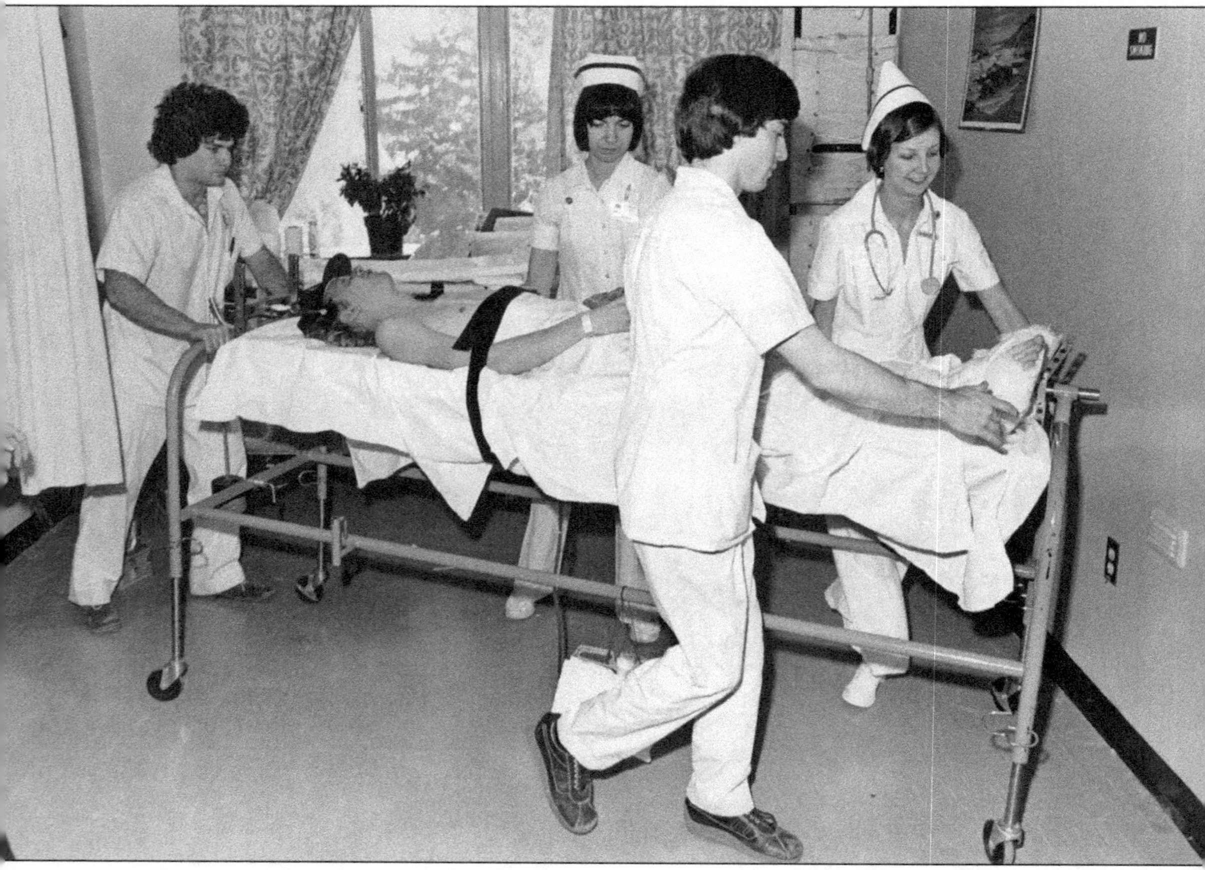

William Landry (left) and other staff move a patient into an intensive care unit during the three-day Blizzard of 1978. The storm dropped four feet of snow on Weymouth; high tides destroyed shorefront homes. A state of emergency was declared. Non-emergency driving was prohibited. Employees lived for a week at the hospital. The Friends of South Shore Hospital gift shop ran out of toothbrushes and toothpaste. The cafeteria ran low on food until it was replenished by the National Guard. Nurses slept wherever they could find a space. Some staff skied to work while one employee walked all night from her home in Hanover, five miles away. Later, civil defense, fire, and police departments, like Abington's, drove staff to work. The staff who bivouacked at the hospital had a lifetime of memories and was proud to put aside personal concern for the good of patients.

Six

Care at Home
With Dignity and Independence

New Englanders were still shoveling out from the Great Blizzard of 1888 that killed 400, when eight women met at Miss Newell's Braintree home. They organized the Philergians for community service and philanthropy.

At the same time, public-spirited women in Weymouth organized the Weymouth Visiting Nurse Association (VNA). Their headquarters, called the Dispensary, was a wooden building in East Weymouth's Jackson Square. It was in 1919 that the Weymouth VNA purchased its first car so that nurse Katherine Dowling Pratt no longer had to use the streetcar to visit patients. Outgrowing the Dispensary, the Weymouth VNA moved to a basement room in the town hall in 1928 and later to the town hall annex.

Visiting Nurse Associations from Braintree, Weymouth, Randolph, Scituate, and Holbrook later combined to become the Visiting Nurse Association of the South Shore. In 1983, the VNA Foundation of the South Shore was formed as the umbrella for the Visiting Nurse Association of the South Shore, Hospice of the South Shore, and Home and Health Resources of the South Shore. Nearly 90,000 home visits were made. Nearly $225,000 in free care was provided. The VNA Foundation formally affiliated with South Shore Hospital in June 1994 and later became a division of the hospital.

Into the 21st century, South Shore Visiting Nurses remains the oldest and the largest home-care agency in the region, making 250,000 home-care visits annually to 7,000 patients in 27 communities. It has 450 employees. It is ranked in the top 25 percent of home-care providers nationally.

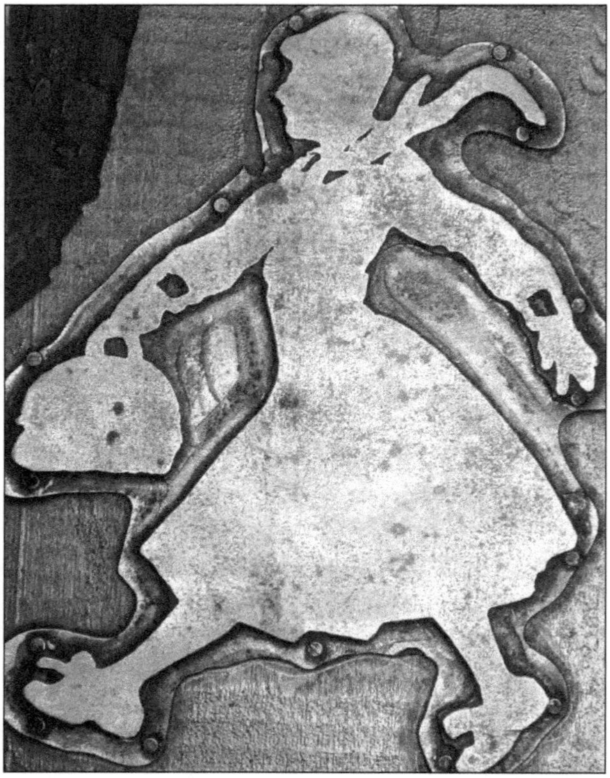

This nurse in stride was the Visiting Nurse Association symbol. Nurses not only cared for the health of their patients, they guided them to more productive lives. Their mission was to "promote health care, prevent disease, provide skilled nursing care, and encourage thrift, self-dependence and industry through friendly advice and sympathy."

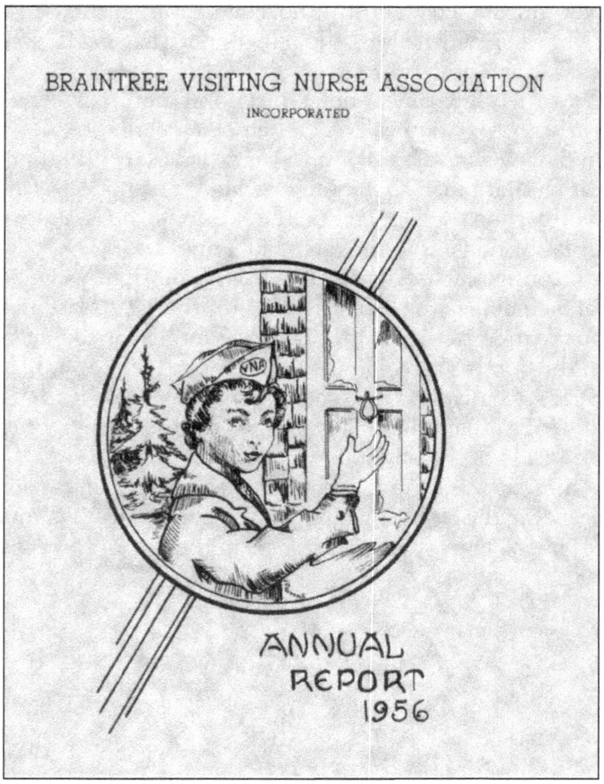

An early Braintree VNA hand-drawn annual report cover portrays nurses in the style of Florence Nightingale. Over the years, home health services grew in stature as professional, humane, and yet economical care. With nurses making 2,000 visits in 1918, an office opened part-time at 109 Railroad Street in Braintree just in time to marshal against the influenza epidemic. By 1921, a supervisor was hired, and the office was open all day.

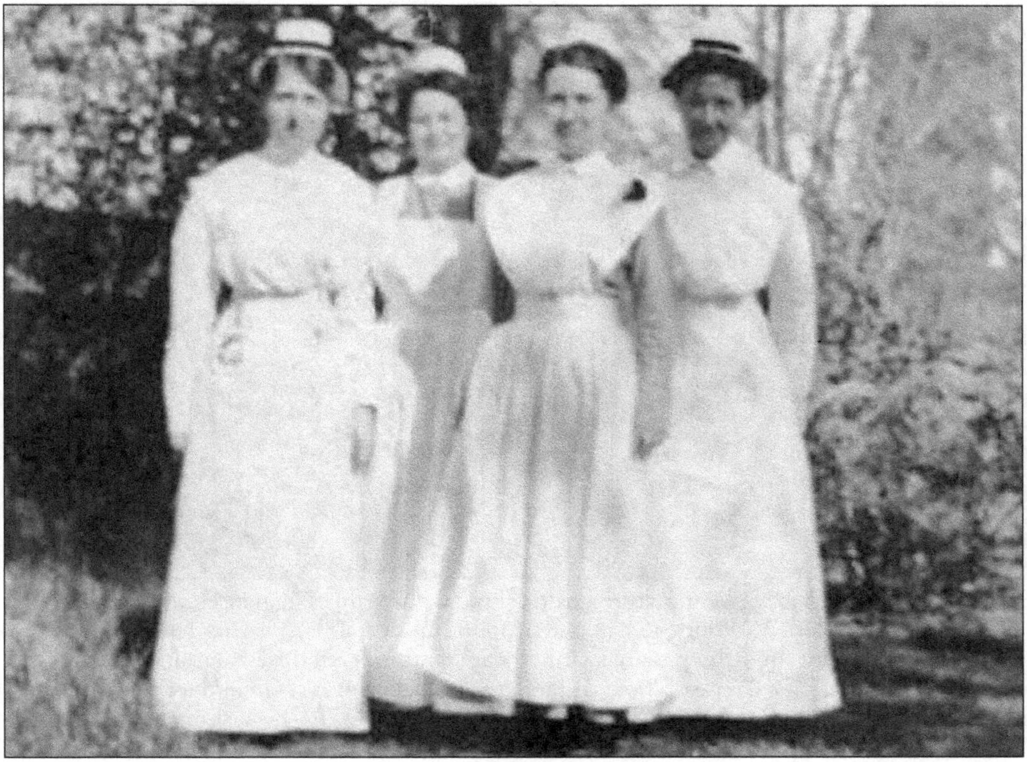

With donations from events, the Braintree Visiting Nurse Association (BVNA) hired its first nurse in October 1911. She was on duty six days a week from 8:00 a.m. to 5:00 p.m. Her one-month paid vacation had to be used "exclusively for rest and recreation." The nurse could be reached by addressing a postcard to P.O. Box 35 or by leaving a telephone number at Torrey's Drug Store in South Braintree. She called there each day before traveling by streetcar to patients' homes. Often, the families needed more than health care, and the society hired a social worker in 1912. In the first year, the nurse and social worker made 1,756 visits, charging from 5¢ to 50¢. In winter, nurses wore long woolen capes. Pictured above are BVNA nurses wearing starched whites in the summer of 1911. At right is an example of the "military style" uniforms of the 1950s.

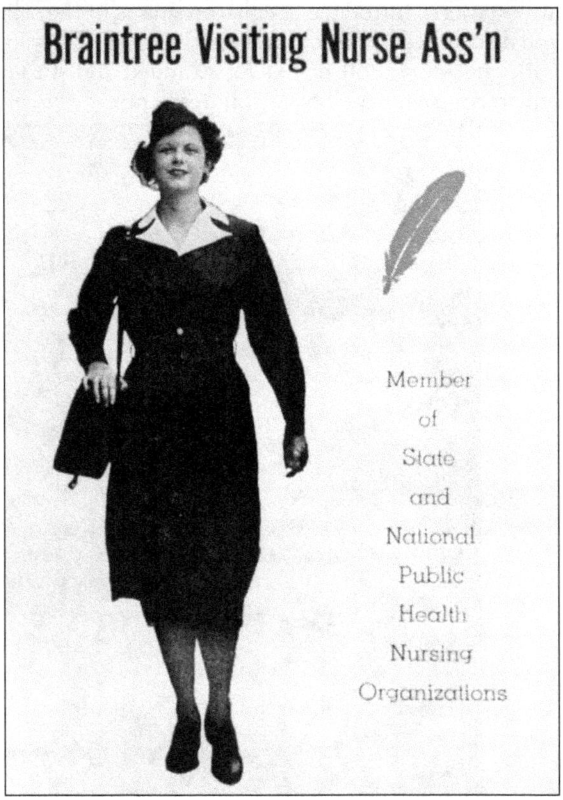
Braintree Visiting Nurse Ass'n
Member
of
State
and
National
Public
Health
Nursing
Organizations

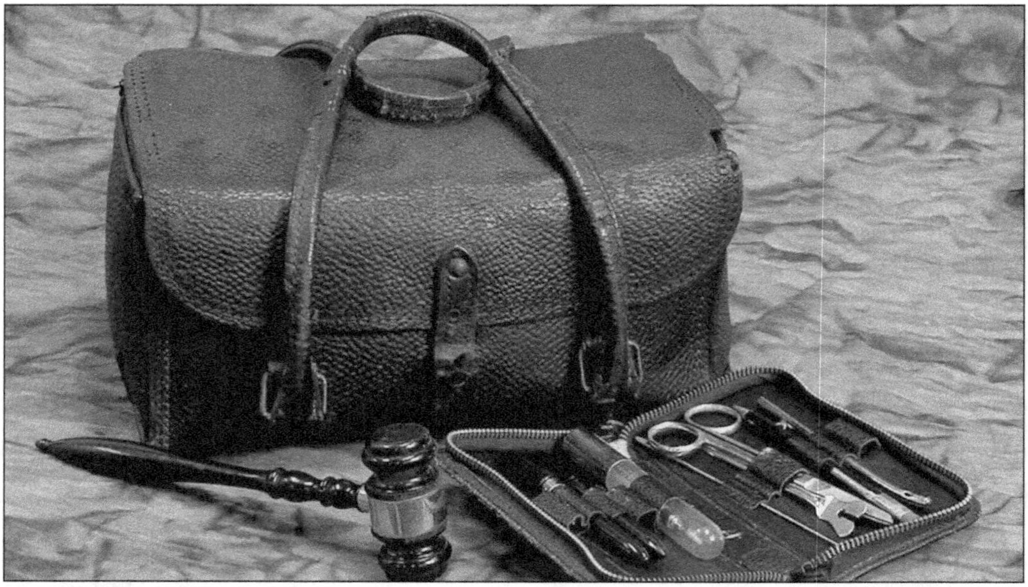

The leather nurse's bag was a miniature health clinic with syringes, bandages, and medications in small glass bottles. Without the equipment found in hospitals, Visiting Nurses had to be creative. They often used the patient's tinned cans and measured steps around the kitchen table for rehabilitation exercises. These ammonia salts (below) were standard for reviving light-headed patients or family members. Medicine was not all that was in the Visiting Nurse's bag. As "overseers of the poor," they sewed layettes, delivered thousands of babies, ran dental clinics and milk stations, introduced health programs in the schools, assisted victims of industrial accidents, and distributed holiday baskets to the needy. They arrived in blizzards and heat waves, delivering milk and Moxie soft drinks for stranded and starving families. Visiting Nurses were often the only recourse for the town's frail residents.

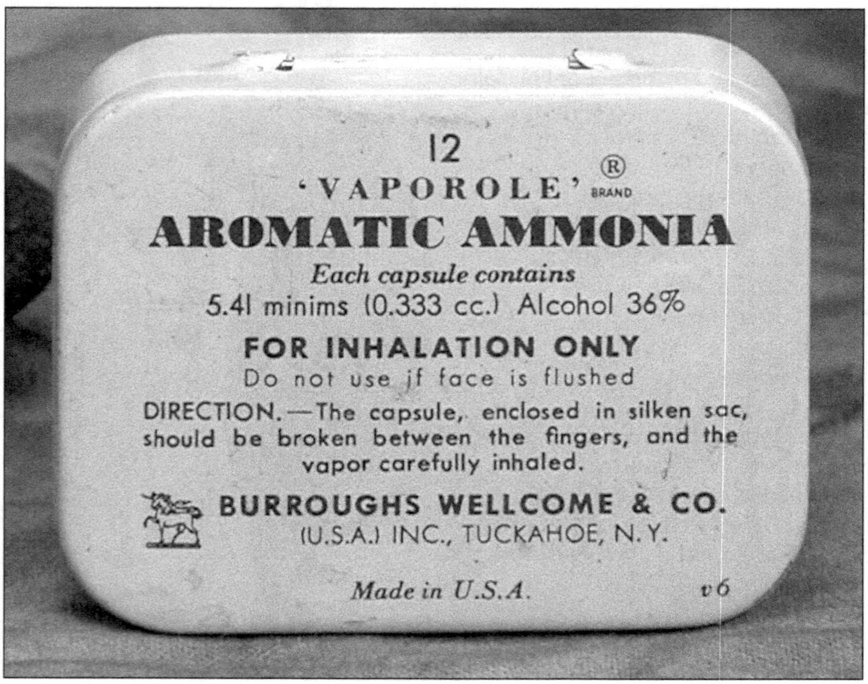

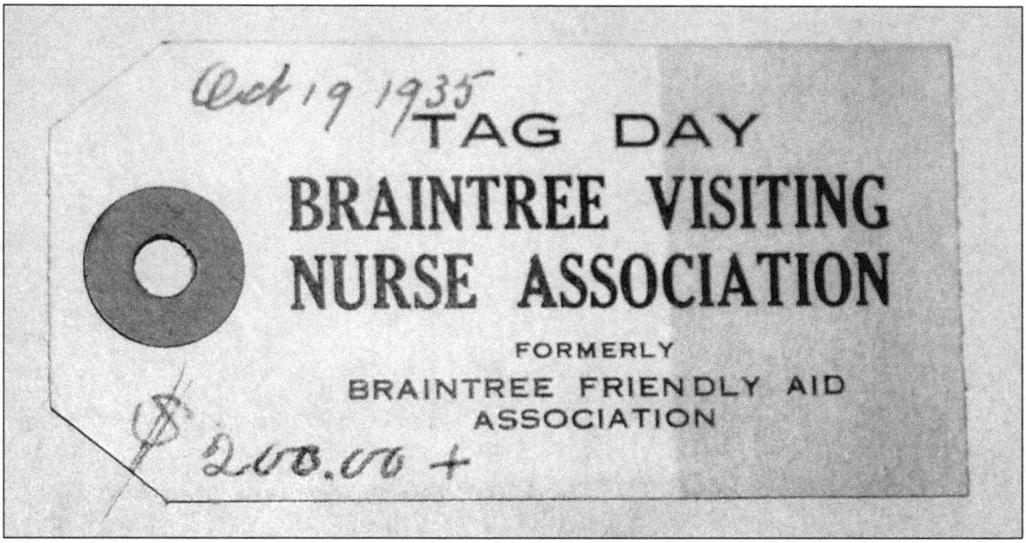
Oct 19 1935
TAG DAY
BRAINTREE VISITING
NURSE ASSOCIATION
FORMERLY
BRAINTREE FRIENDLY AID
ASSOCIATION
$200.00 +

VNAs became adept at fundraising to subsidize care. In a newspaper advertisement for a one-week fundraising appeal in May 1921, the Braintree Friendly Aid Association sought "free-will gifts" to "relieve suffering." In a 1935 Braintree VNA tag sale, an unidentified item was $200, a large amount in the Depression. Another VNA event offered a rare ride around Braintree in an automobile.

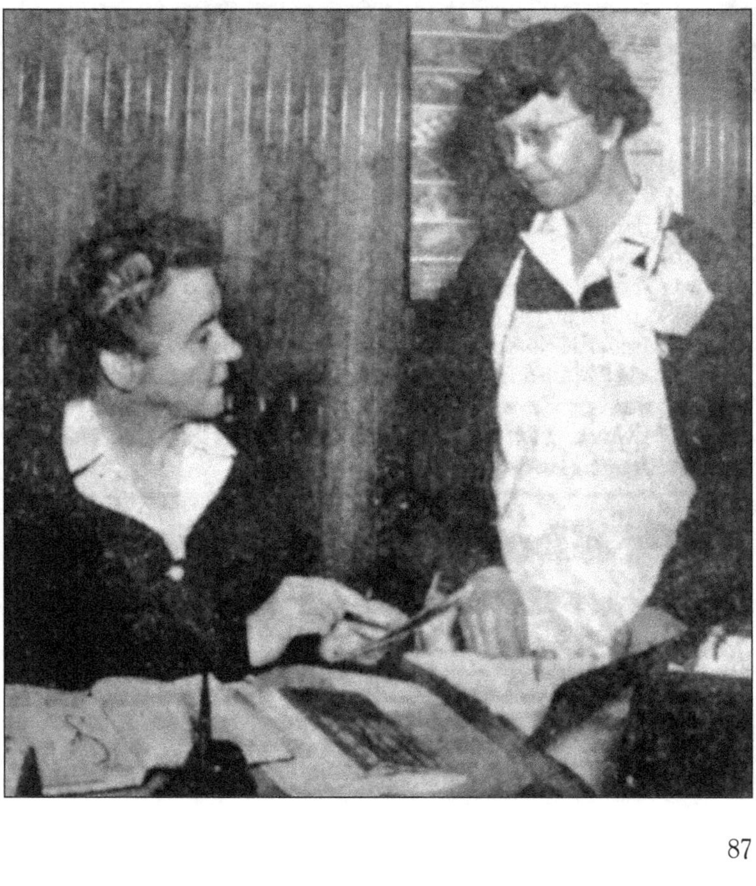

Braintree VNA public health director of staff Catherine Murphy (seated) speaks with nurse Esther Bates before Bates leaves for her daily home visits. Braintree VNA officers continue to meet at All Soul's Church to make all nonclinical decisions. Leaders included Mrs. Eugene Muller, Mrs. Harold Robinson, Mrs. Arthur G. White, Mrs. Edgar Copper, Mrs. E. Curtiss Mower, and Mrs. Ray Worthen.

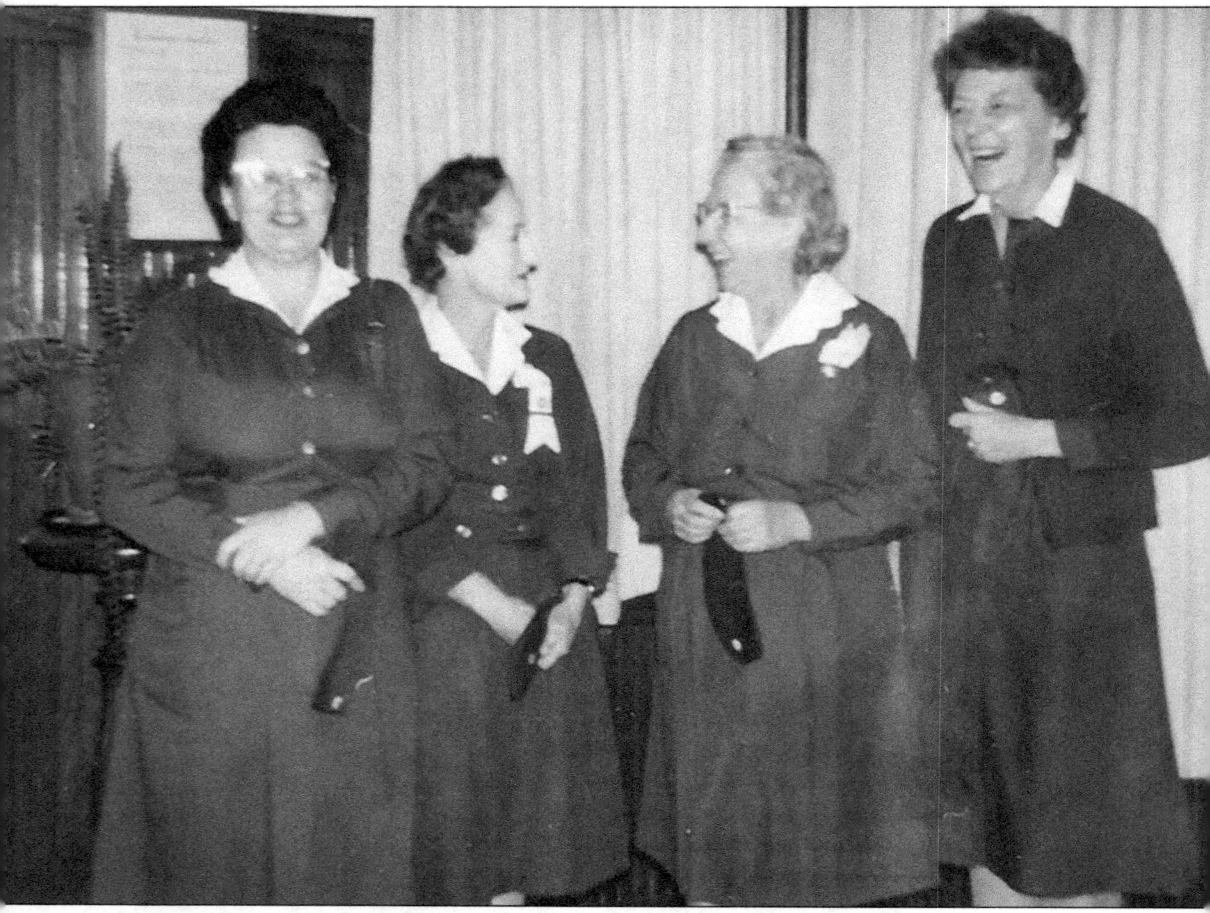

In 1963, Braintree Visiting Nurses, like (from left to right) Ethel Warren, Roancy Horne, Catherine Dunn, and Elizabeth Cropper, made 8,620 visits. Most were made to bed-bound patients, to help new mothers, and to assist patients in managing health conditions. Tuberculosis was still a concern. Nursing visits of an hour or less were $2.50, more than an hour was $3, and an office visit was $1.50. Just over half their visits were fully paid; the rest were partial or free care. Often, the VNAs relied on the towns for support, a lifeline that ended during the Depression. In addition to home visits, the nurses held clinics in local industries and for well children and served as camp and nursery-school nurses. Dr. Arthur Sullivan was medical advisor, assisted by Drs. Luman Woodruff, Robert Ross, and Robert Clancy. The nurses worked from 648 Washington Street in Braintree every day except Sunday.

The Massachusetts House of Representatives commended the Braintree VNA on its 60th anniversary in 1971. With the proclamation are VNA board president Marjorie Bryant (left) and Alva Dow, who started the organization and served as a president and board member for over 50 years. This was no longer a part-time endeavor with a nurse traveling by streetcar. Home care required highly skilled nurses, and Braintree VNA incorporated professional staff education. The same degree of expertise was also required in the boardroom, and the need was met by business executives and professionals actively involved in operations. Leading the board in those pivotal years were Mildred Cotton, Marjorie Bryant (whose family owned Lauriat's bookstores), and Donald Olson, Braintree Savings Bank president and the first male on the VNA Board. South Shore Visiting Nurses is now the oldest and largest home-care agency in the region.

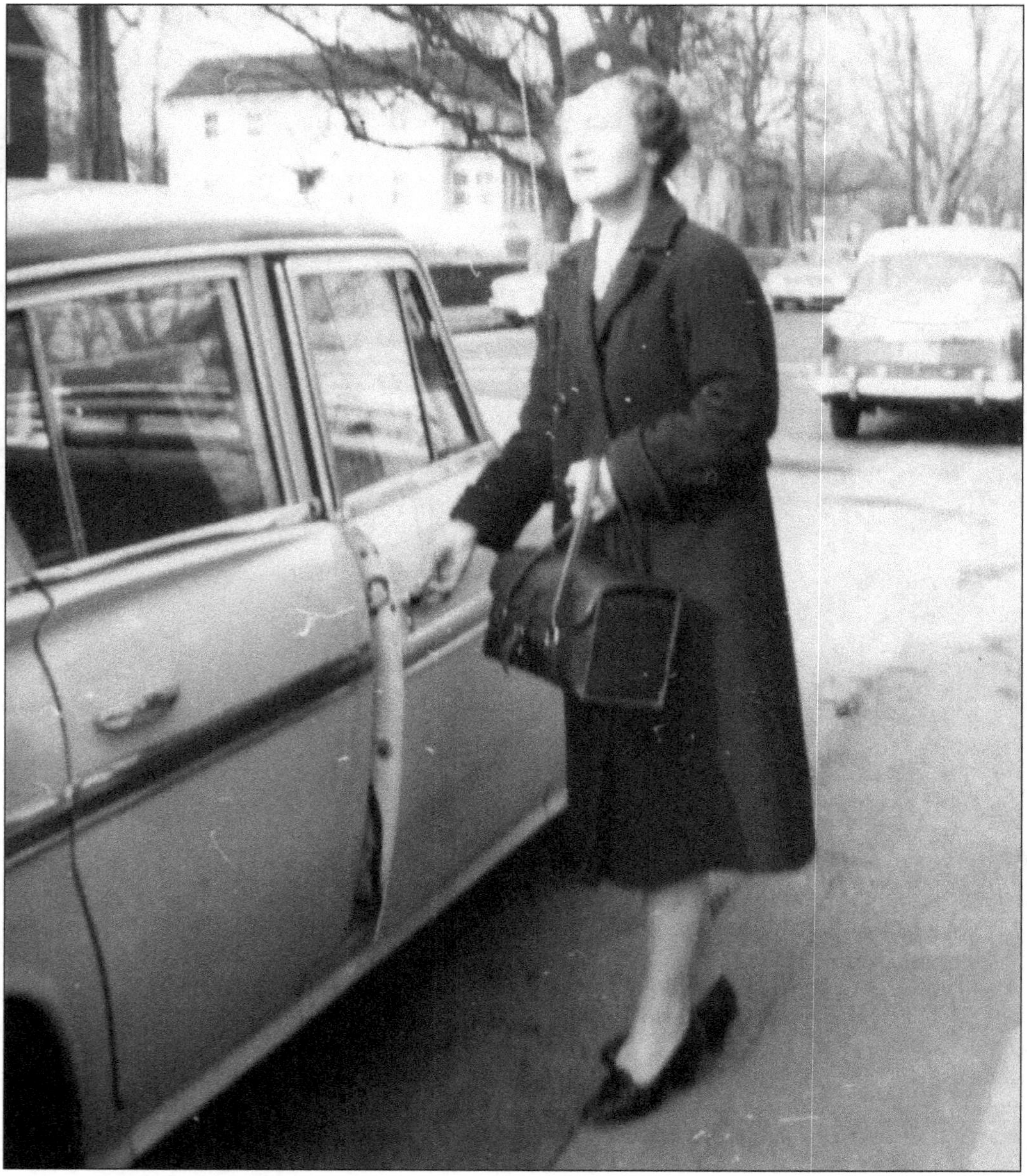

In the early decades of the 20th century, Visiting Nurses traveled to more distant patients' homes by streetcar and trolley. It was not surprising that a fundraising advertisement in 1921 listed "the little car" as the nurses' top aid, even before the telephone and supplies closet. This photograph of an unidentified Braintree Visiting Nurse is likely from the 1950s.

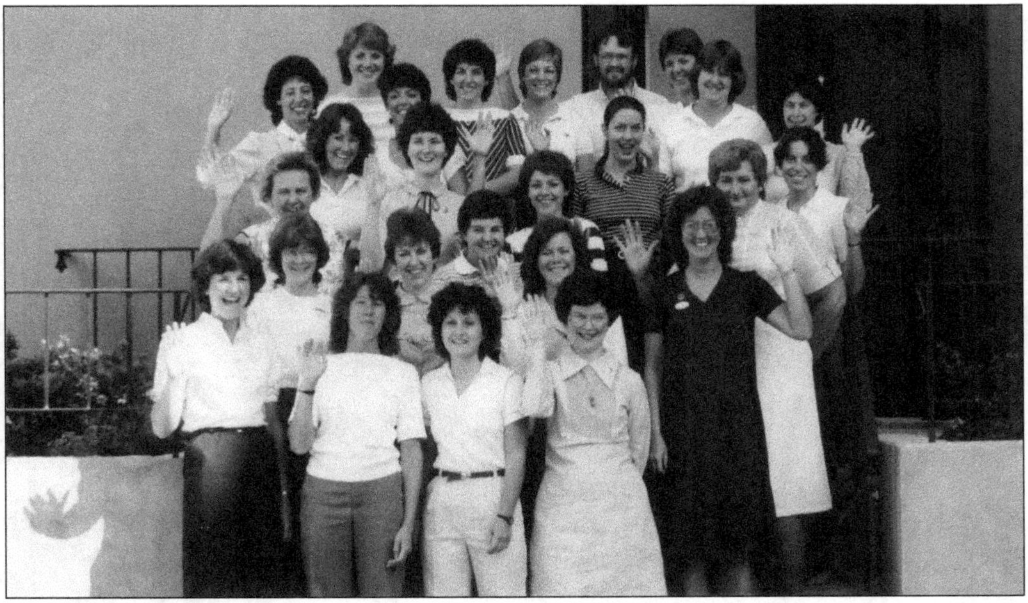

Visiting Nurses pause before traveling to patients' homes from then-new headquarters at 400 Franklin Street, Braintree. South Shore Visiting Nurse Association was comprised of the previously town-specific VNAs in Braintree, Holbrook, Randolph, Scituate, and Weymouth. They developed specialized nursing teams to care for the growing number of patients with more complex conditions.

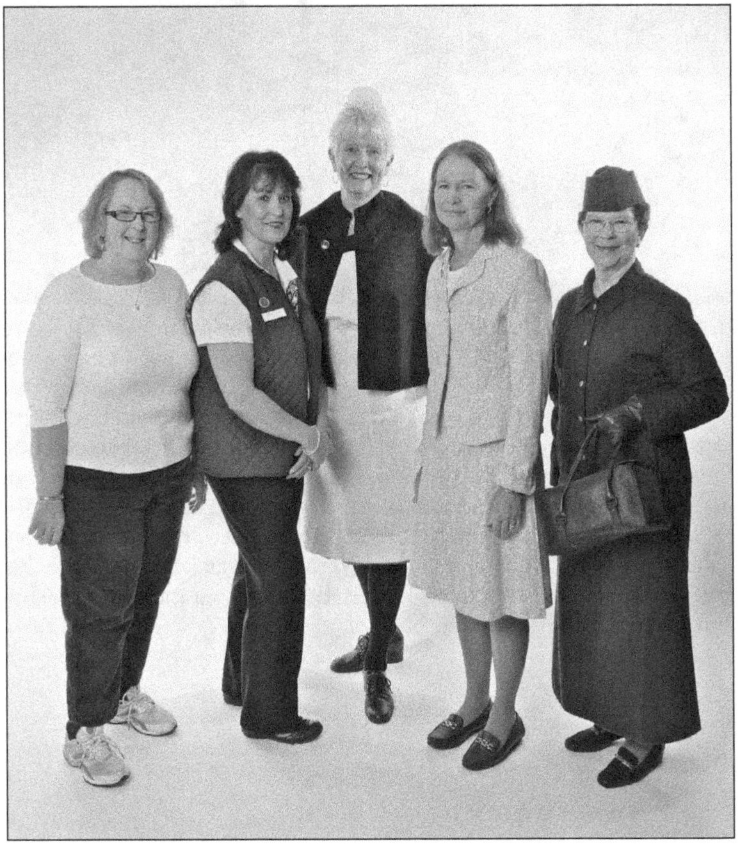

Appearing in vintage Visiting Nurse uniforms are, from left to right, Kathleen Maitland (2000), Joyce Cox (1990s), Jane Shea (in her 1960s nursing student uniform), Patricia Smith (1980s), and Judy Charron (1920s). To protect patients' privacy, nurses wear everyday clothing. With Medicare and Medicaid coverage for home visits, the nurses treat more complex conditions and have developed specialty teams of highly skilled nurses and therapists.

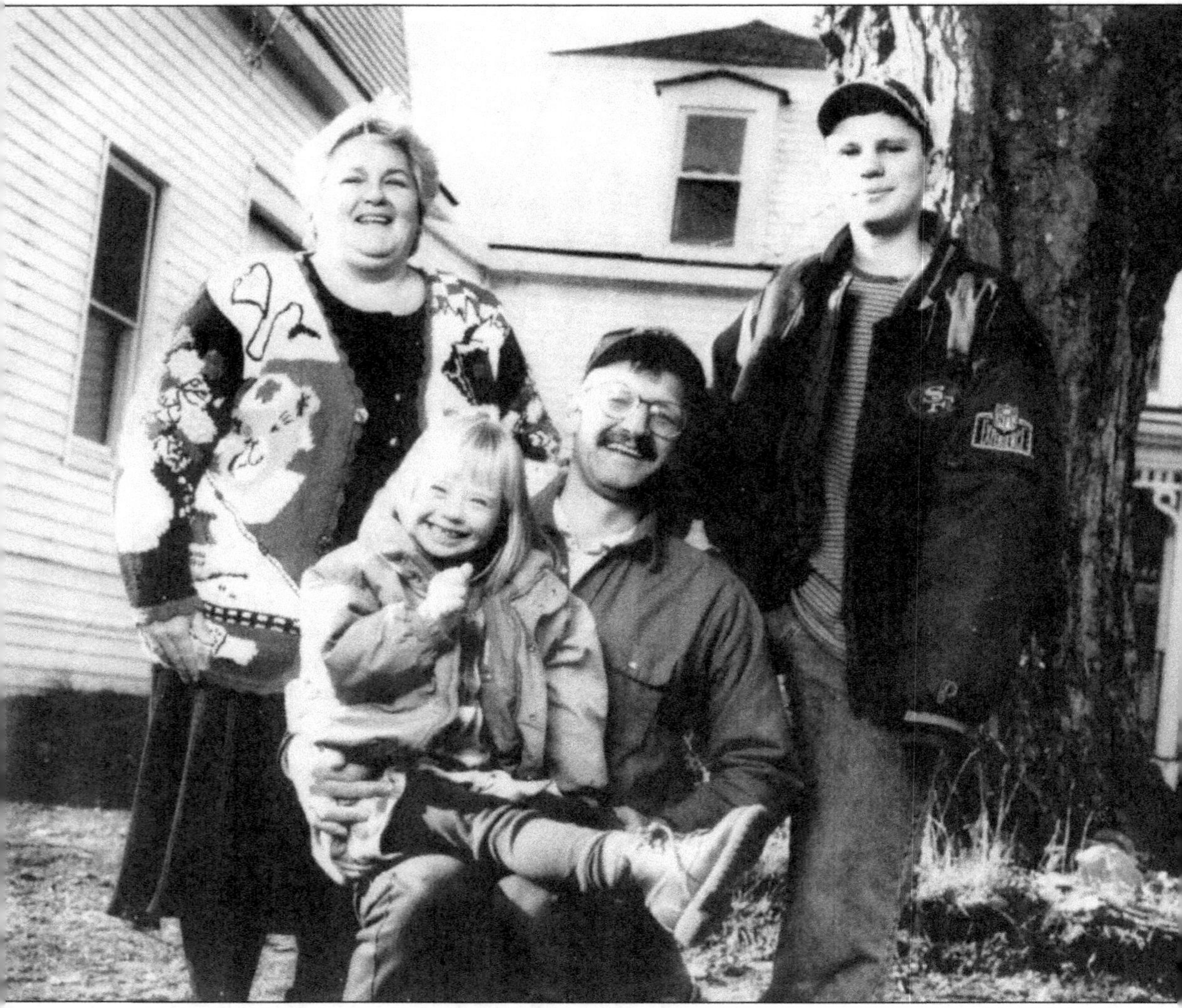

In October 1996, Jack Tamulevich's life changed forever. A tree surgeon, he was removing a tree damaged by a storm when the removal rope snapped and he was thrown on the front steps of the house. With broken hips, knee, pelvis, ribs, elbow, and wrist, plus a fractured skull, the physicians did not expect him to live. After four months in hospitals, Jack returned home unable to walk or even feed himself. South Shore Visiting Nurse Association physical and occupational therapists, social workers, and home health aides all helped him regain his independence. To treat his severe infection, intravenous nurse specialist Ann Cashman visited him daily to administer IV medications. "Ann not only treated my infections, she lifted my spirits," Jack said gratefully. "She's pure sunlight." Thanks to the team and Jack's persistence, he was able to return to work and walk without assistance. In this 1998 photograph, Ann Cashman, left, joins Jack, center, and his children Rachel and Samuel.

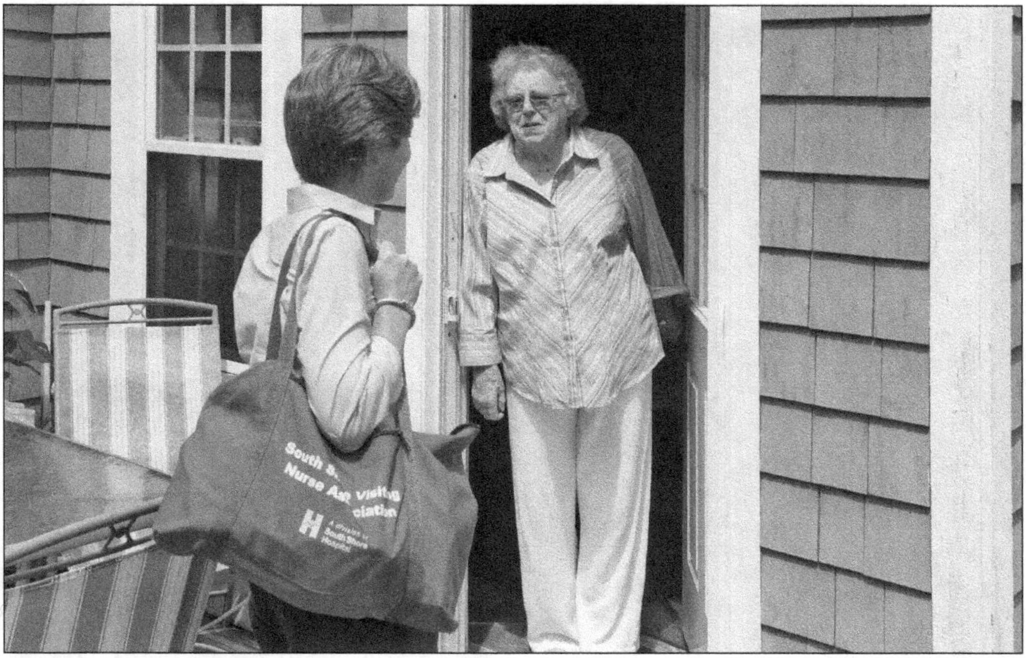

Home-care nurse Nancy Daly is welcomed by Doris Hogan during one of the 150,000 visits that the VNA makes annually in 27 communities. With baby boomers aging, more people 85 and older, and a cultural preference against instituting elders, more families rely on home-care services. At the same time, reimbursements are being cut, increasing the reliance on donations.

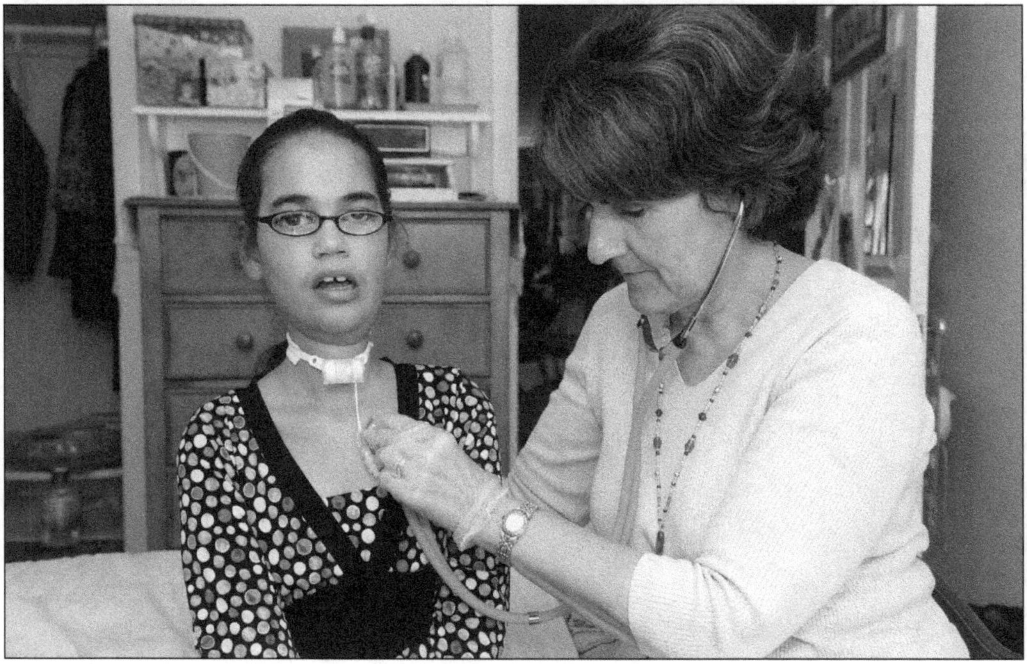

The hospital's home-care division helps patients transition from the hospital to home. As more procedures are performed in homes, patients can be discharged confident that they will receive expert care outside the hospital walls. Nurse Lynn MacDonald flushes Nicole Coulimore's tracheotomy. The VNA cares for increasingly more pediatric patients with complex health conditions.

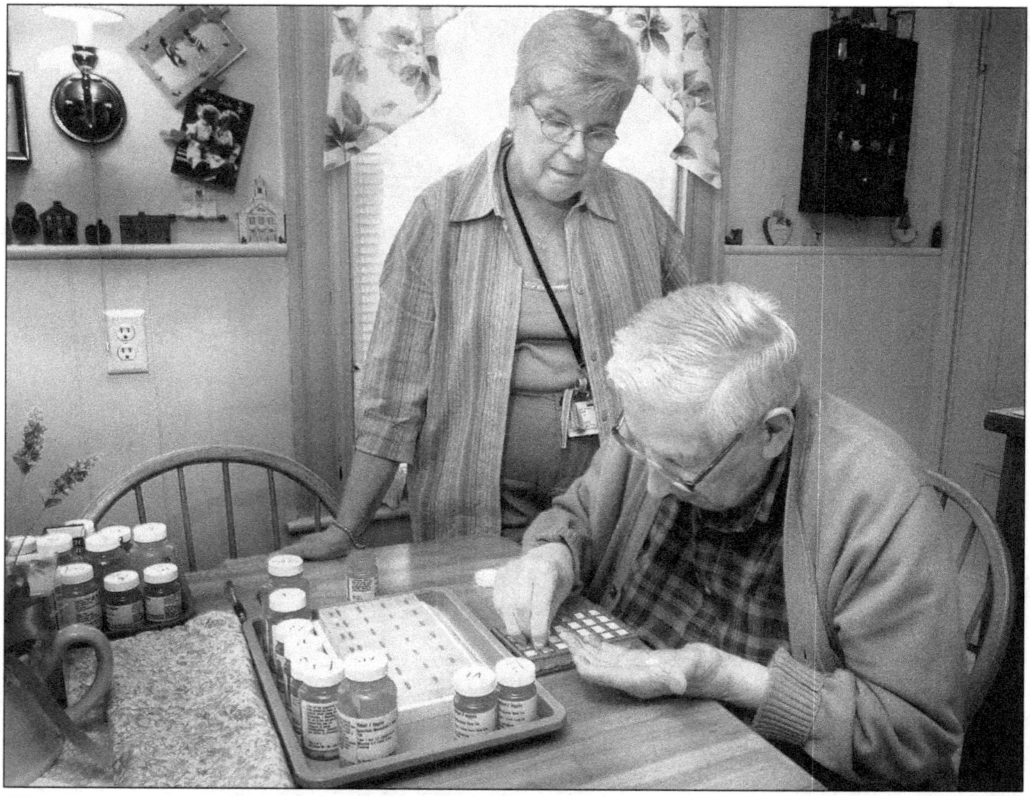

When elders have multiple and complex conditions, they often have to manage many medications. Nurses, like Jane Keefe, and aides help ensure that patients like Robert Higgins take the right medications at the right time, so the drugs work properly and do not cause a toxic reaction. This assistance is invaluable for elders living alone.

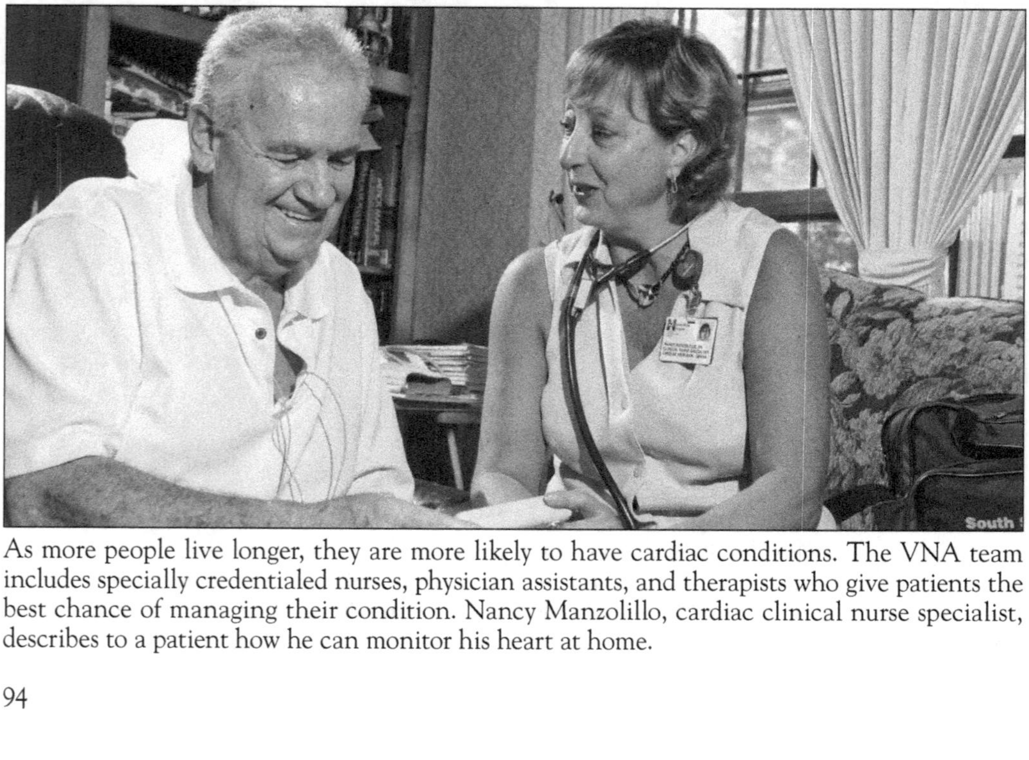

As more people live longer, they are more likely to have cardiac conditions. The VNA team includes specially credentialed nurses, physician assistants, and therapists who give patients the best chance of managing their condition. Nancy Manzolillo, cardiac clinical nurse specialist, describes to a patient how he can monitor his heart at home.

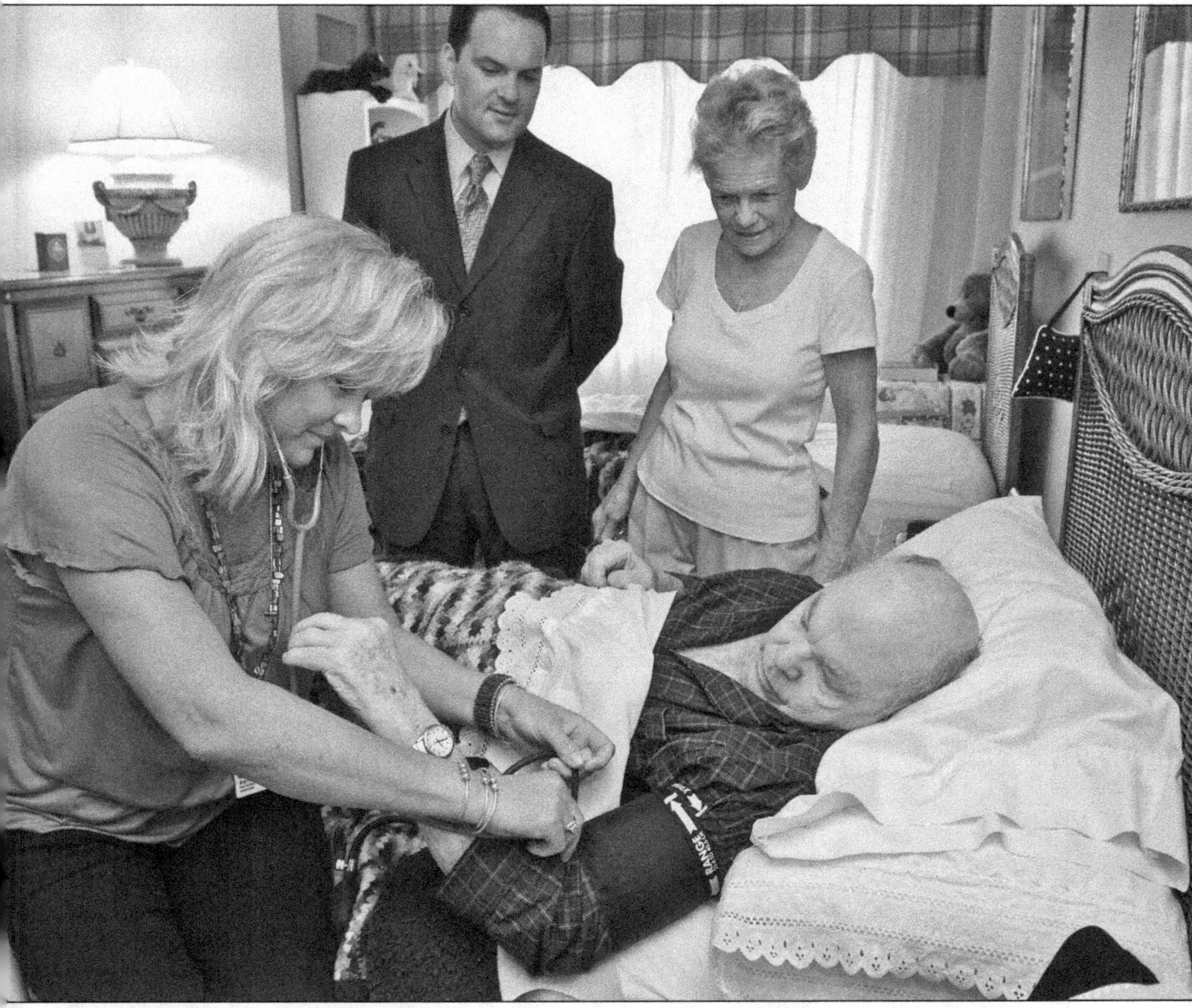

Hospice patient James Ireland welcomes Garrett Bradley, state representative, into his house to show how hospice care reduced his pain and enabled him to spend his remaining time at home with loved ones. With Ireland are his wife and the hospice nurse Patricia Corliss (left). Hospice of the South Shore is the largest hospice program in the region. The hospice team is comprised of physicians, nurses, physical and occupational therapists, and social workers, coordinating to make the patient as comfortable as possible when a cure is unlikely. Hospice also provides spiritual support to those patients who request it. Many volunteers help patients live as fully as they can by engaging them in favorite activities and giving respite to their caretakers. Because hospice cares for the family as well as the patient, bereavement support is available for grieving families. Although provided at the end of life, hospice care is an affirmation of the dignity of the patient.

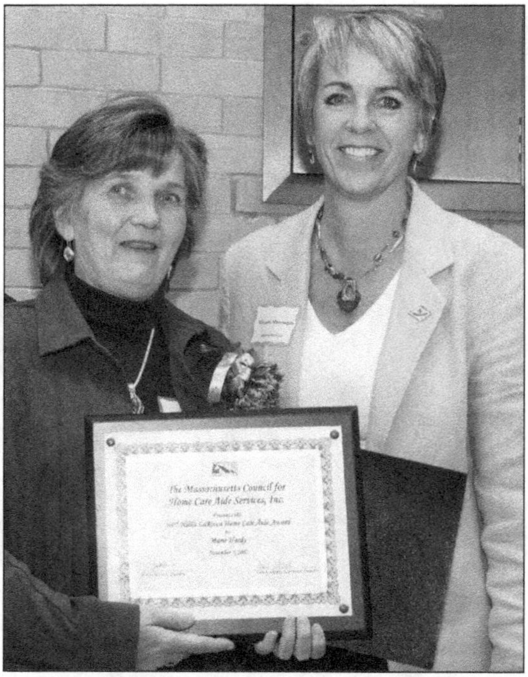

When Marie Hardy (left) won the Hilda LaRocca Award as top home health aide in the commonwealth, she joined other honored aides Rosemary Parkman, Pat Scopa, and Phillip Dwyer. Muriel Oakman, of Braintree, wrote the regulations that created the professional home health aide in Massachusetts. Oakman later was president of South Shore VNA. With Hardy is Marianne Mastrangelo, of the American Red Cross.

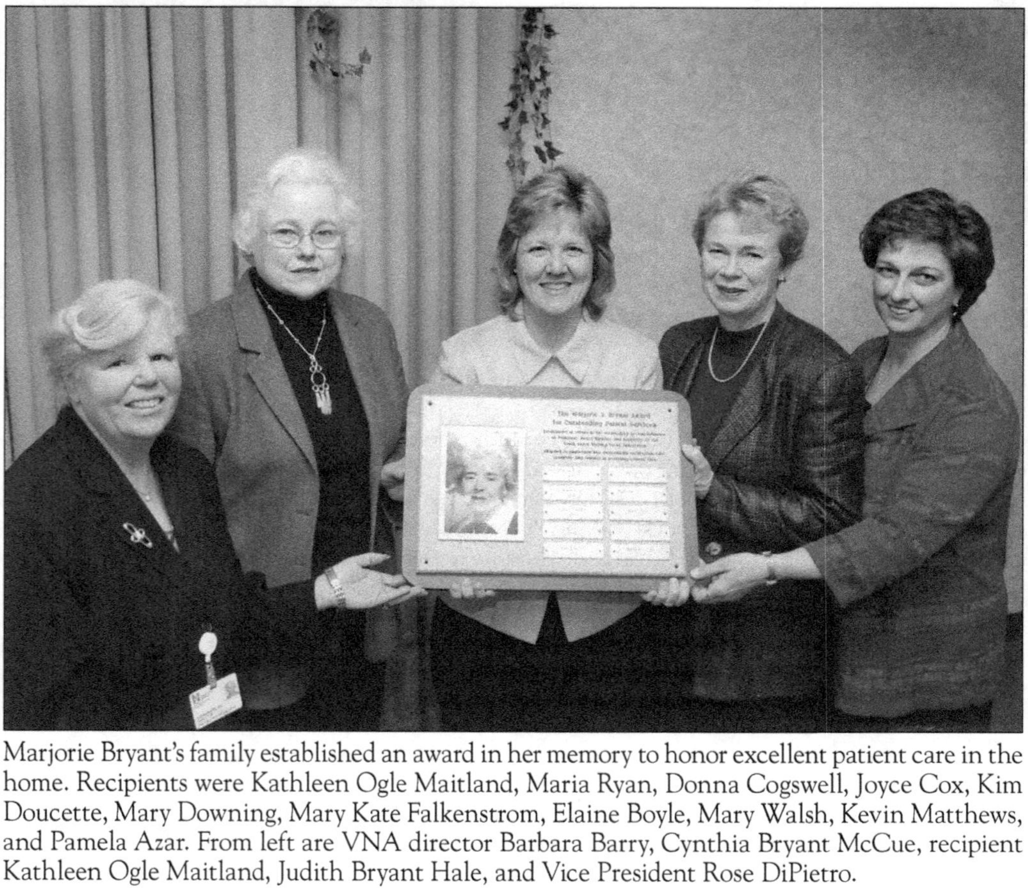

Marjorie Bryant's family established an award in her memory to honor excellent patient care in the home. Recipients were Kathleen Ogle Maitland, Maria Ryan, Donna Cogswell, Joyce Cox, Kim Doucette, Mary Downing, Mary Kate Falkenstrom, Elaine Boyle, Mary Walsh, Kevin Matthews, and Pamela Azar. From left are VNA director Barbara Barry, Cynthia Bryant McCue, recipient Kathleen Ogle Maitland, Judith Bryant Hale, and Vice President Rose DiPietro.

Seven

Friends & Volunteers

"Cheerful Deeds of Kindness and Service"

When Florence Hatch formed the Women's Guild soon after the hospital was founded, its goal was to improve "the stays of patients and the working conditions of staff." Women of great energy, they held teas, parties, and balls. Each year, May Emerson and her production committee cut more than three football-field lengths of fabric and sewed thousands of towels, gowns, sheets, diapers, dressings, and even hot-water bottle covers.

With World War II labor shortages and a waiting list for beds, board president Carleton Barnes envisioned "a different type of service—that of the volunteer worker—helping us carry on some of the non-professional duties in caring for the sick."

And so was born the Friends of South Shore Hospital with 187 members each paying $1. While still producing soft goods and decorating the hospital, their focus was fundraising and volunteering.

The Friends have contributed millions to improve patient care, established five scholarships, and recruited thousands of hospital supporters. In 2010, the Friends was formally enfolded into the hospital and now has 2,000 members in 14 states.

Florence Howe Hatch and Alice Barnes served as presidents of the Women's Guild. Friends presidents were Edith French, Mrs. George Anderson, Marjorie Benedict, Mrs. Laurence Jasper, Mrs. Knutson, Mrs. Arthur Chubbuck, Ruth W. Wilkie, Mabel Melvin, Mrs. William Seabury, Mrs. Woodworth Murray, Ruth Asher, Veronica Oman, Mrs. William, Hunnewell Beal, Mrs. James Giles, Jane Phillips, Nancy Buttrick, Ruth Chambers, Barbara Romeo, Betty Wylie, Barbara MacSwan, Ruth Asher, Barbara Hamer, Bridget Blasser, Louise Connelly, Joy McKee, Lucy Kalaijian, Mildred Cotton, Marie Goodwin, Susan Fillipi, Lois Bisson, Ellen Scott Garvey, Donna Stearns, Geraldine Thomson, and Tina Kosinski.

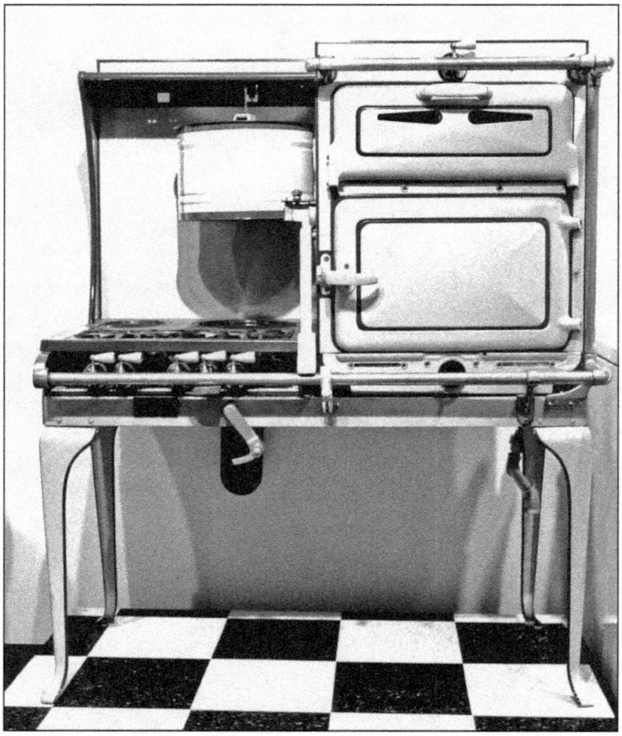

This 1930s stove was similar to the one that the Women's Guild donated to the hospital. Within a decade of the founding of the hospital, the guild raised enough to replace the Reed Mansion's aging kitchen appliances. The members also sewed all the tray cloths and donated the china service. For decades, they delivered ice cream and cake to patients at Thanksgiving and Christmas. (Courtesy of Myrna Walsh.)

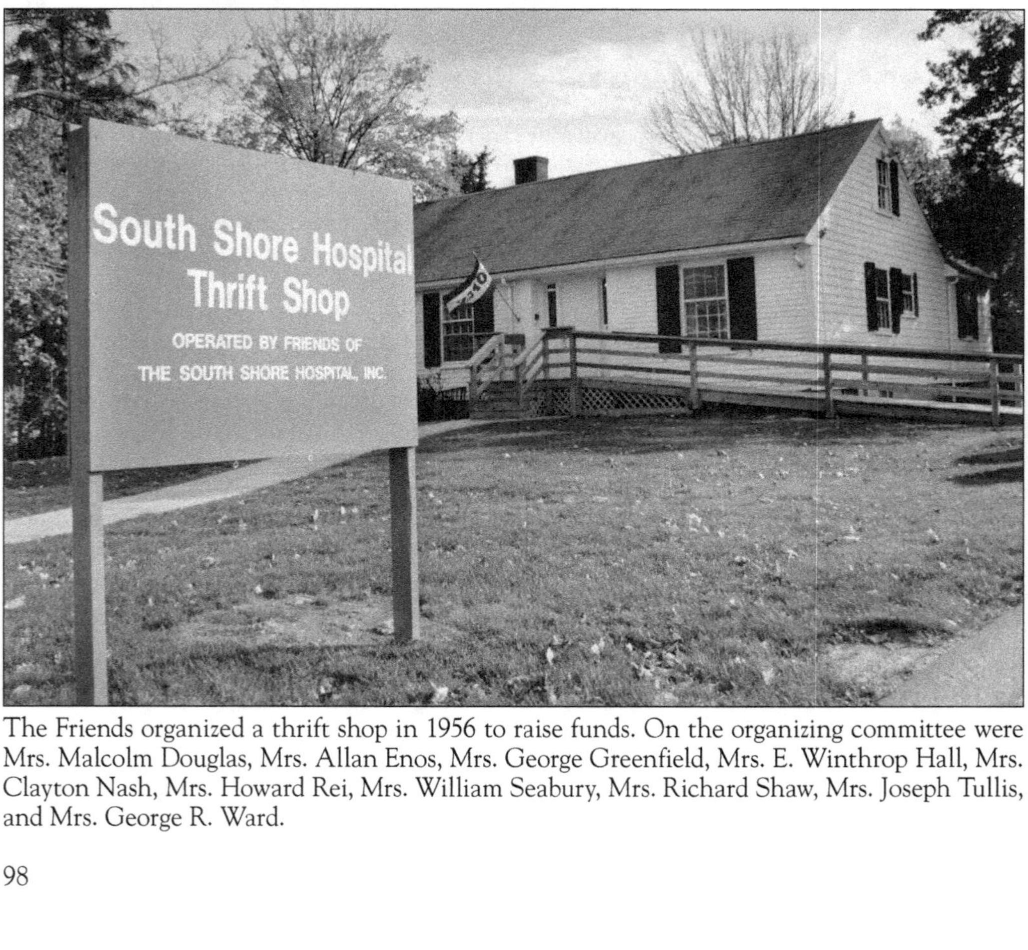
South Shore Hospital
Thrift Shop
OPERATED BY FRIENDS OF
THE SOUTH SHORE HOSPITAL, INC.

The Friends organized a thrift shop in 1956 to raise funds. On the organizing committee were Mrs. Malcolm Douglas, Mrs. Allan Enos, Mrs. George Greenfield, Mrs. E. Winthrop Hall, Mrs. Clayton Nash, Mrs. Howard Rei, Mrs. William Seabury, Mrs. Richard Shaw, Mrs. Joseph Tullis, and Mrs. George R. Ward.

Mrs. William Hunnewell Beal presided over the Friends from 1967 to 1968 when sales from the shop reached a record at that time of $21,700. The Friends paid its $40,000 pledge, bought a new sewing machine for the linen room and curtains for the boardroom and cafeteria. Friends continued to generously provide equipment as the hospital built new facilities.

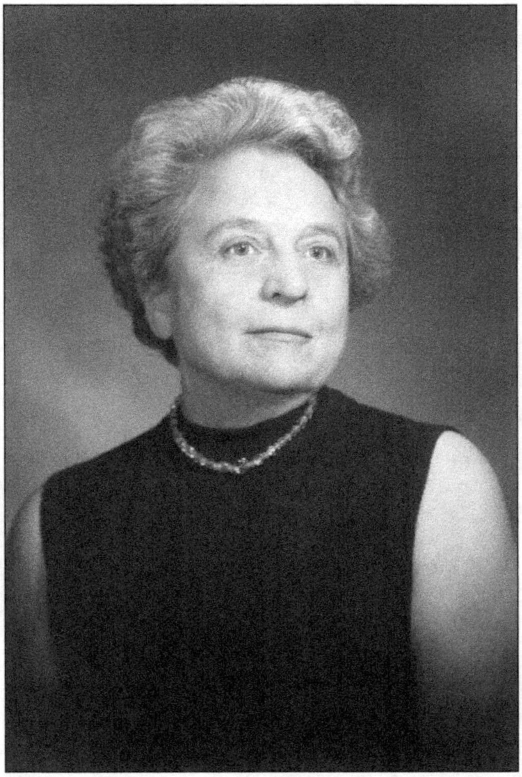

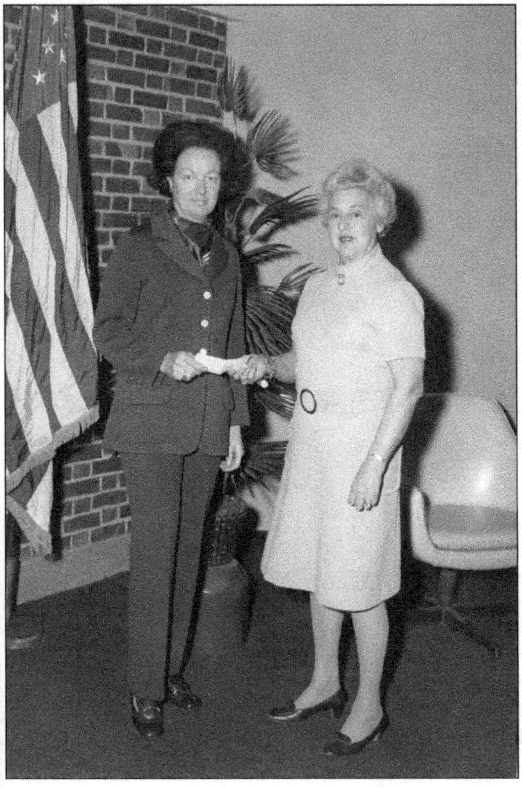

Joan Roche (left) hands a check from fundraising to Friends president Ruth Chambers in 1971. The Friends had 700 members. Henry Hoffman summed up the Friends' contribution years before when he noted, "They are compassionate people, concerned about other people, and they go all out. They give more than 100 percent to make this a pleasant, ongoing operation."

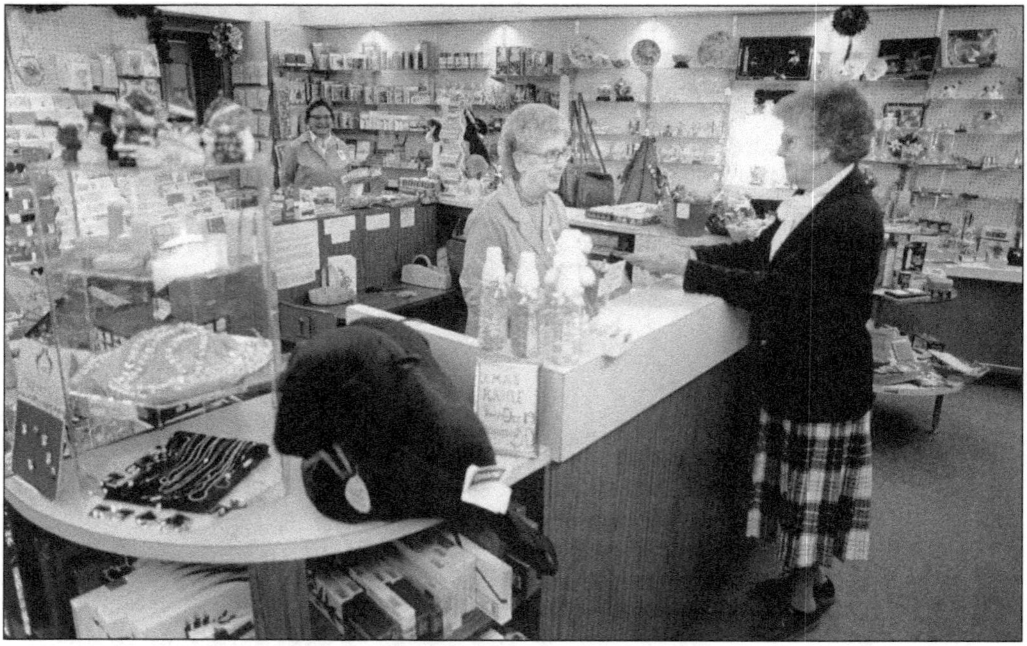

From left to right, Beatrice Jenkins, Margaret Knox, and Eleanor Cormach staff the Friendly Shop. The Friends opened the shop in 1949 with $175. The profit grew from $131 in the first two months to $1,219 five years later. The Friendly Shop sells small gifts and sundries. The Cottage Shop, first in Columbian Square and later on Fogg Road, sells high-quality clothing, home decor items, and gifts.

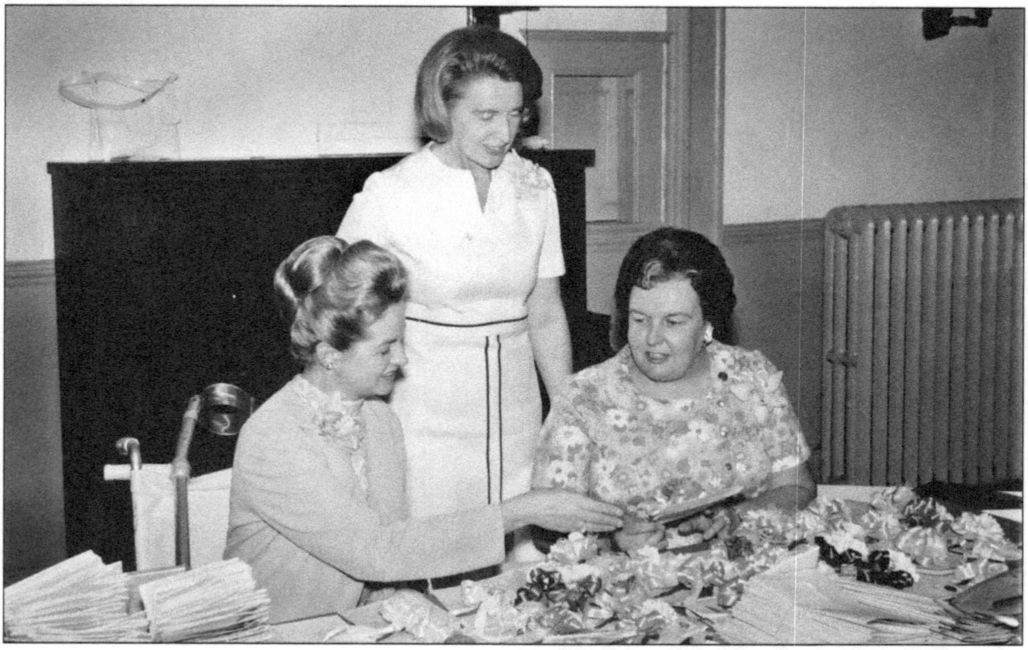

From left to right, an unidentified Friend, Jane Philips (standing), and Nancy Buttrick work on a Friends project. Jane Phillips was Friends president and later became the first female hospital board chair. A mathematics teacher in Abington, Philips received membership in the newly formed Friends as a wedding shower gift from her future mother-in-law, Isabel Phillips, a longtime Women's Guild member. After World War II, the Women's Guild became the Friends of South Shore Hospital.

Past presidents at the Friends 50th anniversary in 1997 pose with hospital president David Hannan. From left to right are Louise Connolly, Bridget Blasser, Hannan, Nancy Buttrick, Barbara Hamer, Veronica Oman, and Joy McKee. Far from the stereotypical "blue-haired ladies," Friends are a fundraising powerhouse. Traditional women's events, like teas, were replaced with golf tournaments, croquet matches, runs, strolls, and walks that attract all ages and raise more than $1 million annually.

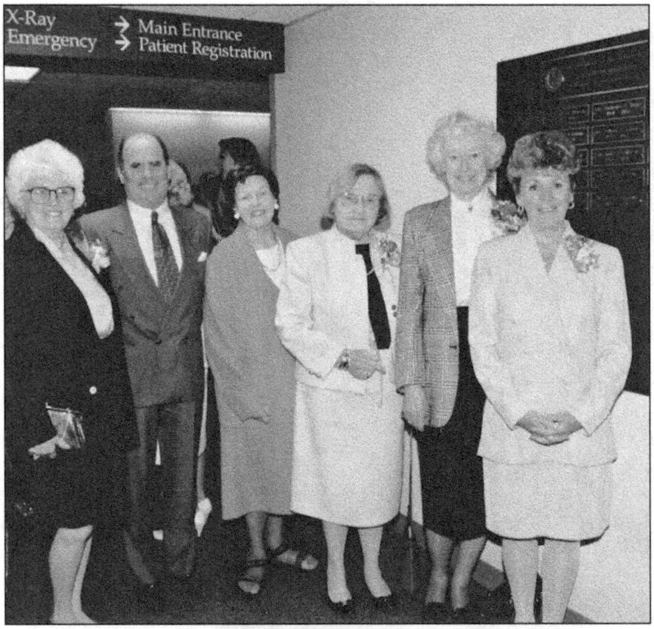

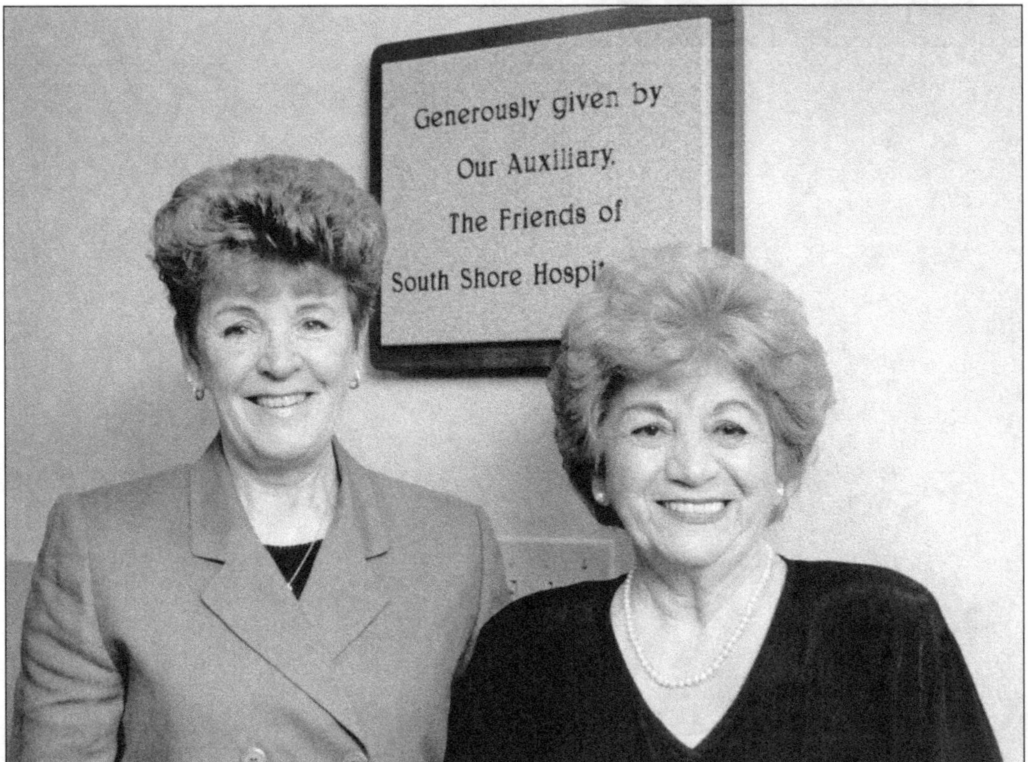

Outgoing Friends president Joy McKee (left) and incoming president Lucy Kalaijian fulfilled a $500,000 pledge in 1997. Since the early days when the main activity of the Women's Guild was sewing thousands of items for Weymouth Hospital and arranging flowers for patients, the Friends has expanded to 2,000 members organized into committees with close ties to specific clinical programs, such as cardiac and pediatrics.

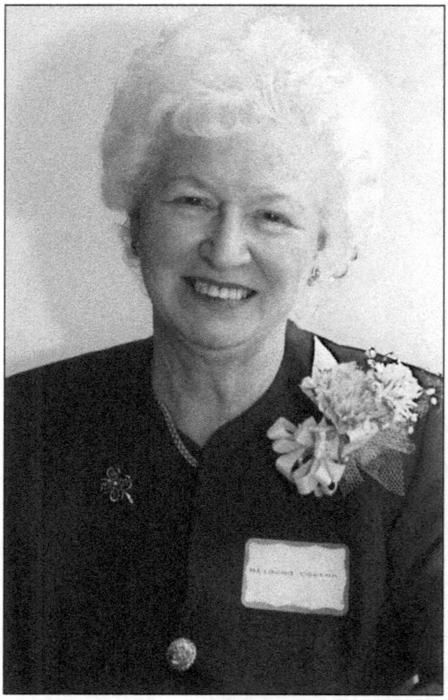

South Shore VNA president Mildred Cotton helped develop sound financial practices while coping with rapid growth. Cotton later was president of the Friends and vice chair of the hospital's Foundation during a period of enormous growth. A longtime member of the Philergians, a charitable organization that established Braintree VNA, Cotton was known for her gracious manner, compassion, and tireless energy.

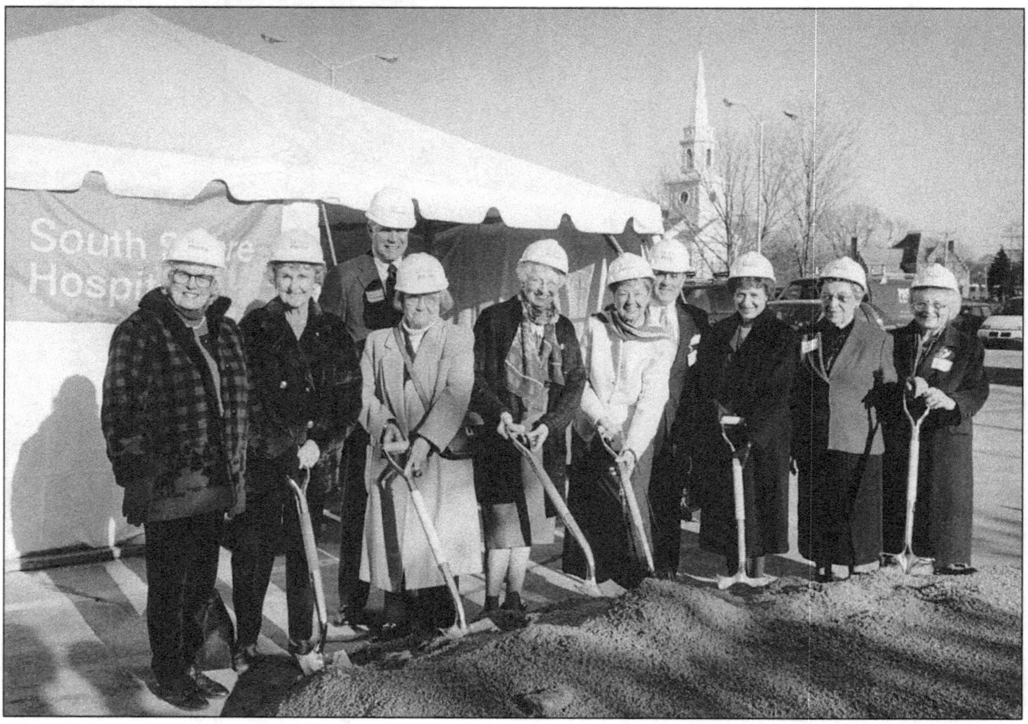

The Friends were a major contributor to the new emergency department, which would become one of the largest and busiest in the commonwealth. At the 1999 groundbreaking ceremony are, from left to right, Bridget Blasser, Louise Johnson, Paul MacElhiney (chairman of the hospital board), Barbara Hamer, Mildred Cotton, Yvonne McGrory, David Hannan (president and chief executive officer), Constance Libardoni, Marie Goodwin, and Nancy Nicosia.

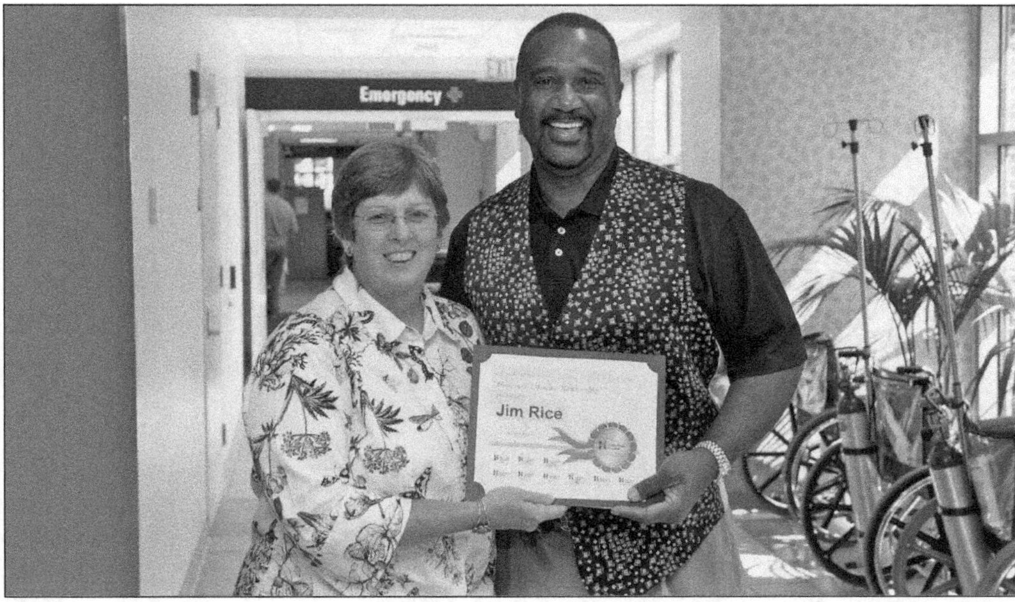

Red Sox baseball Hall of Famer Jim Rice became an honorary Friend during a hospital visit. Welcoming Rice is Friends president Geraldine Thomson. Rice joins other honorary Friends, including First Lady Barbara Bush, Red Sox pitcher Tim Wakefield, astronaut Michael Mullane, news anchors Heather Unruh and Lisa Hughes, captain of the 1980 gold-medal US hockey team Mike Eruzione, and other high achievers.

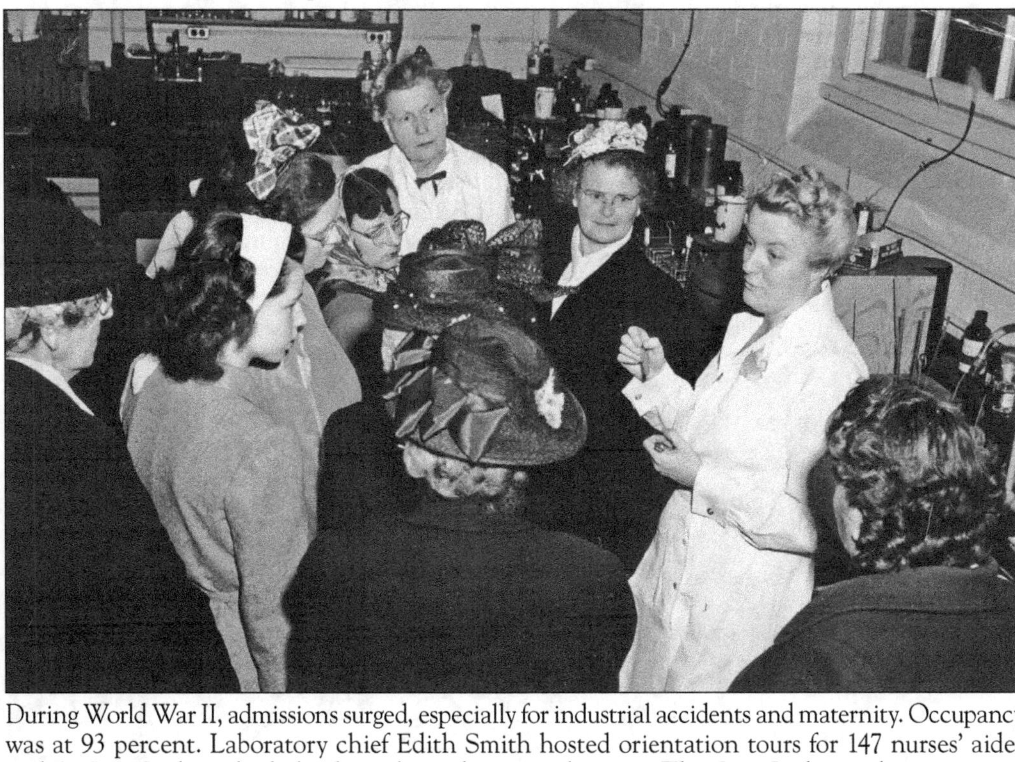

During World War II, admissions surged, especially for industrial accidents and maternity. Occupancy was at 93 percent. Laboratory chief Edith Smith hosted orientation tours for 147 nurses' aides and 58 Gray Ladies who helped to relieve the nurse shortage. The Gray Ladies, volunteers, were named for the gray dresses and veils they wore when first organized by the Red Cross.

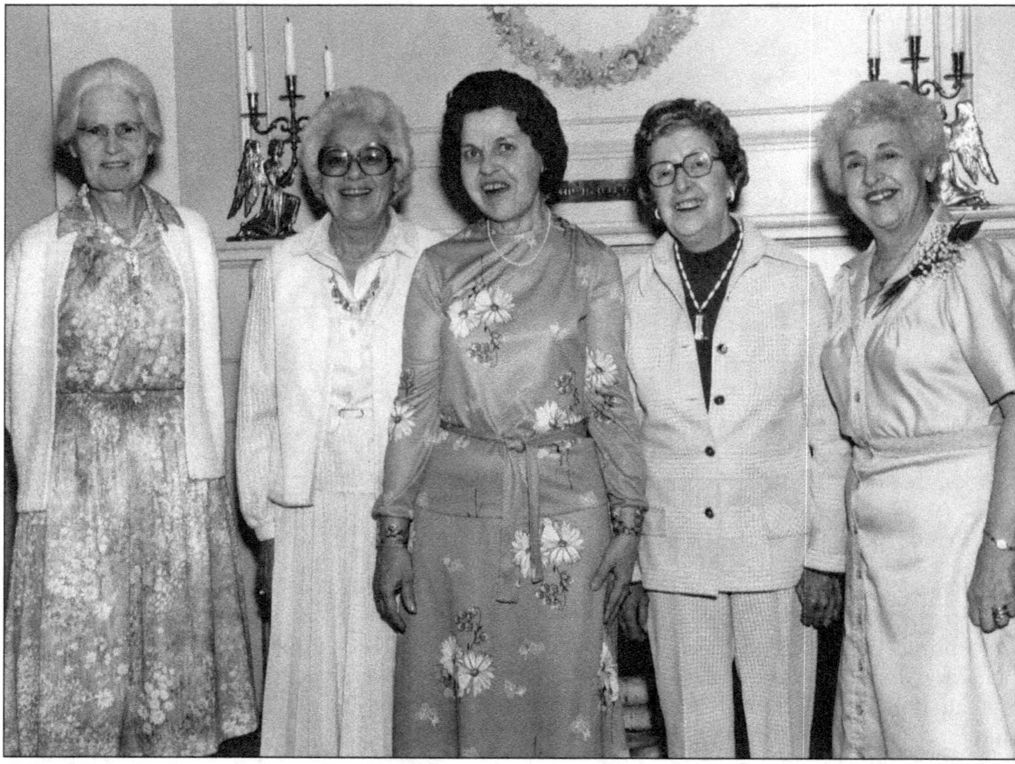

A handful of volunteers contributed 769 hours in just two months when the hospital was founded in 1922. In 10 years, the number exploded as 657 volunteers in "cherry red" smocks gave 25,000 hours. They read to children, maintained a 2,000-book library, arranged flowers, worked as secretaries, and staffed the reception desk. During the severe nurse shortage of World War II, retired nurses volunteered for bedside care. Volunteers were organized under the Women's Guild, then the Friends, and finally as a hospital department. In 1978, the hospital honored 129 volunteers who gave 81,800 hours, an "inestimable amount of financial savings for the hospital." Above, among those who gave more than 5,000 hours each are, from left to right, Thelma Putney, Ruth Asher, Ellen Wennberg, Gertrude Sullivan, and Ruth Chambers. Below, top volunteers in the 1990s are honored. Currently, the hospital's 600 volunteers donate about 90,000 hours a year, the equivalent of $1.7 million annually.

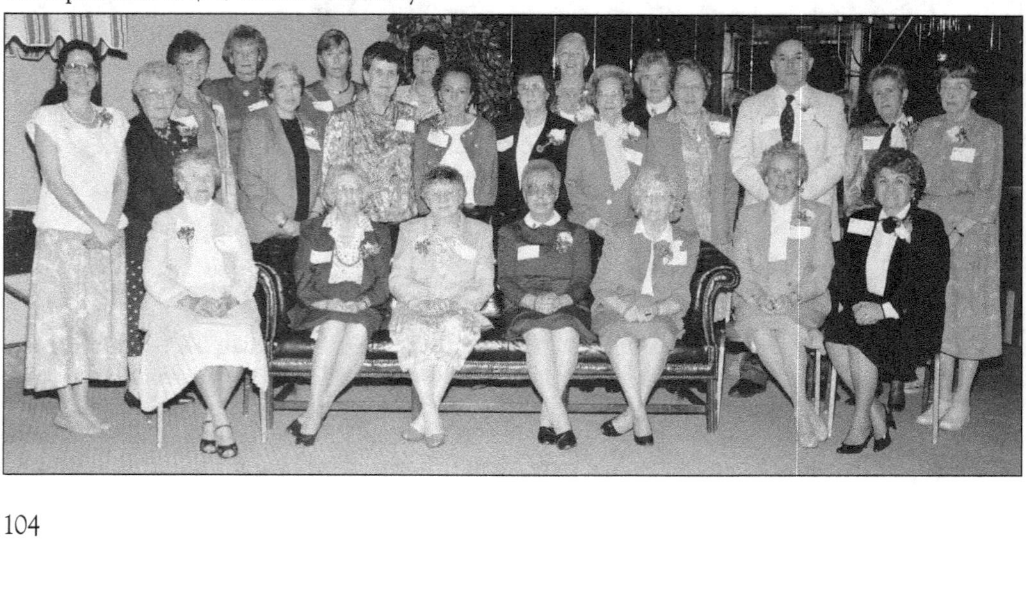

Eight

Philanthropy
"Name Can Live in Usefulness"

South Shore Hospital was founded on two noble but seemingly conflicting standards: no patient would be turned away for inability to pay, and the hospital would be self-sufficient. Adding further financial pressure was the cost of constructing 14 new buildings or major additions at times of daunting deficits caused by charity care, unpaid patient bills, and below-cost reimbursements from health insurers, Medicare, and Medicaid.

According to the 1930 annual report: "The Hospital must be ready to serve any hour of the day or night, which means expensive equipment must be constantly maintained in operating condition as well as a sufficient and competent staff of nurses and operatives always available for duty. These things cost money." Philanthropy was and is the safety net.

Alonzo Newbert donated the first gift of six months of interest on the Reed Mansion's mortgage. In its first decade, the hospital received $143,405 in donations. Trustees personally donated thousands when charity care overwhelmed the hospital budget.

Faced with enormous financial pressure in the 1940s, the trustees reminded the public that "a name can live in usefulness" by annually publishing a wish list. Requests ranged from $30,000 for working capital so that "necessities of patient care may be paid promptly" to $3.40 for a teapot.

Over the decades, the hospital became the charity of choice in southeastern Massachusetts. Since its inception in 1990, the Foundation, now called South Shore Hospital Charitable Foundation, has raised almost $100 million.

Its chairs have been C. Herbert Emilson, Robert Deininger, Bruce Avery, John Doody, David Drohan, Elena Kirkiles, Dr. Philip O'Sullivan, Christopher Oddleifson, and Thomas McCarthy.

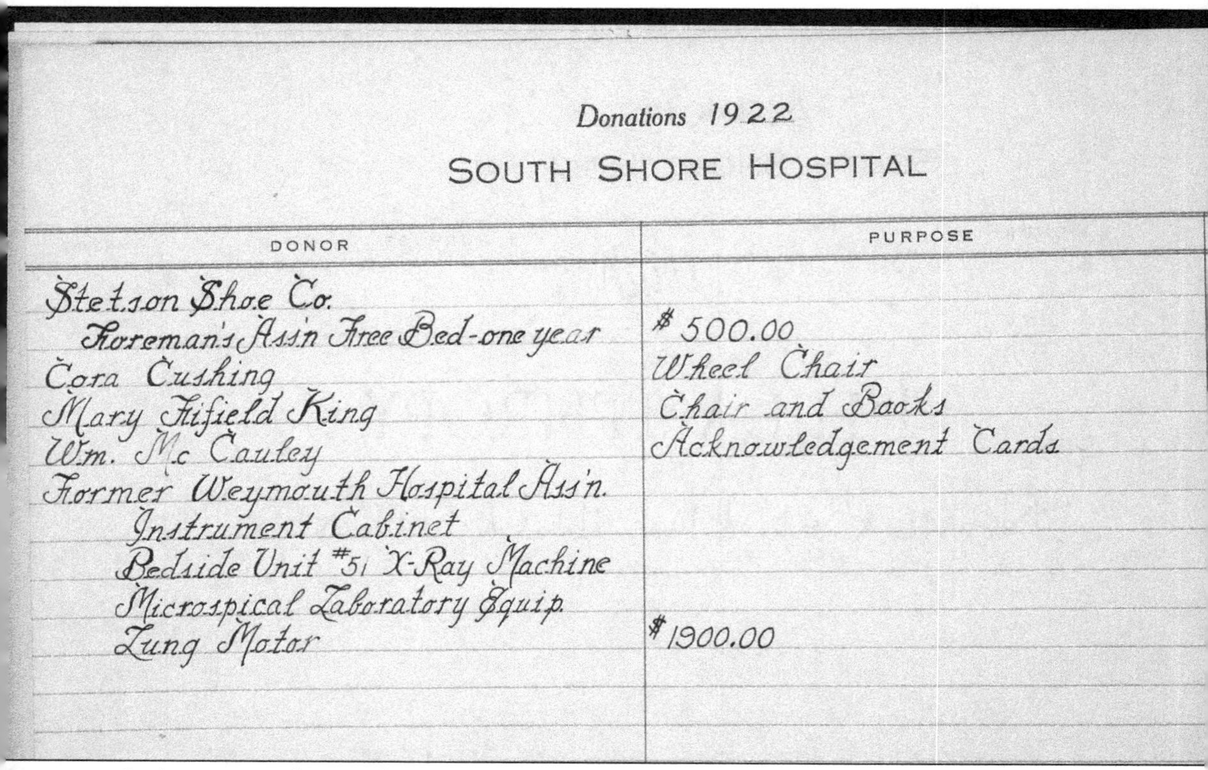

Donations 1922

SOUTH SHORE HOSPITAL

DONOR	PURPOSE
Stetson Shoe Co.	
Foreman's Ass'n Free Bed-one year	$500.00
Cora Cushing	Wheel Chair
Mary Fifield King	Chair and Books
Wm. Mc Cauley	Acknowledgement Cards
Former Weymouth Hospital Ass'n.	
Instrument Cabinet	
Bedside Unit #51 X-Ray Machine	
Microspical Laboratory Equip.	
Lung Motor	$1900.00

Ledger entries show enthusiastic support. In 1922, Stetson Shoe Company donated $1,000, the first of many donations. The former Weymouth Hospital Association, a cottage hospital that had closed by 1922, donated equipment and furnishings worth $1,900. Stetson Shoe Company's management and foremen donated $500 for a free-care bed. (The hospital's original bylaws stipulated that a person or business could reserve a bed and choose who could use it without charge for a year.) Almon Raymond made the first significant gift of $10,000 in honor of his parents when the Reed Mansion proved too small. A few years later, the medical staff paid the $14,000 still owed on the Administration Building, freeing scarce capital for patient care. To help pay for the West Wing, physicians also "taxed" themselves: $5 for each patient admitted and a percentage of charges for procedures. Tonsillectomies, then $35 plus $5 for anesthesia, required a $3 donation. Physicians also paid the balance when the hospital completed the Center Building loan from the government.

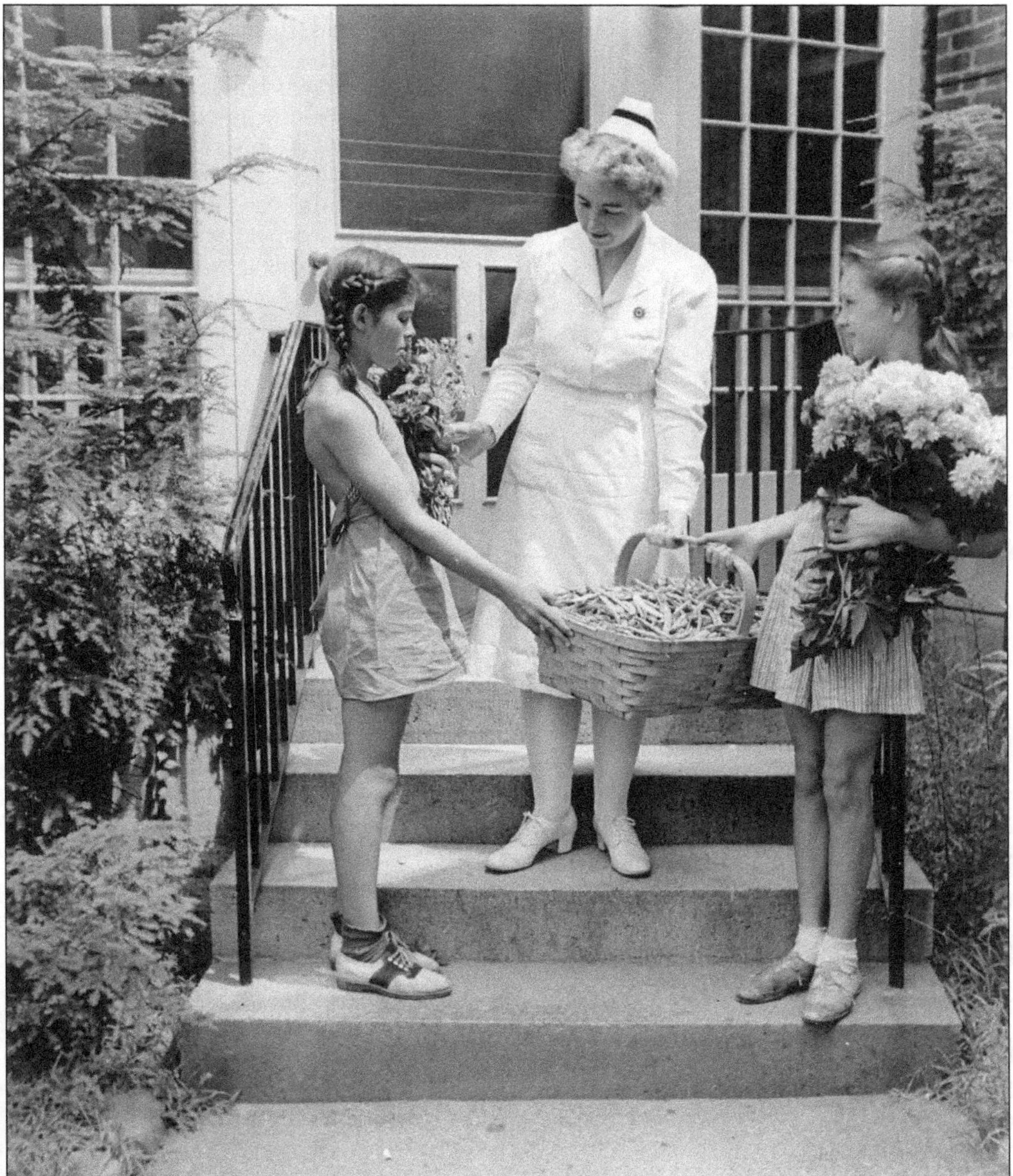

Donation Days began in the Depression and continued through the war years. Children brought homegrown vegetables and preserves to school, which were then delivered to the hospital in Alvin Hollis Company trucks. In 1930, the community donated $350 worth of food, about $5,000 in current consumer prices. The donations helped the hospital stretch its thin reserves when food was rationed during World War II, occupancy was at 93 percent, many patients did not pay their hospital bills, and reimbursements from towns and Blue Cross were uncertain. These community donations represented more than vegetables and fruits. They were continued proof of a close and sustained relationship between grateful residents and the hospital. It is the basis of fundraising to this day. Pearl Hastay in her starched white uniform greets Sally Hurst, left, and Ann Campbell, both from Blanchard Road, who donated vegetables from their Central Street victory garden in 1940. (Photograph by William Rittase.)

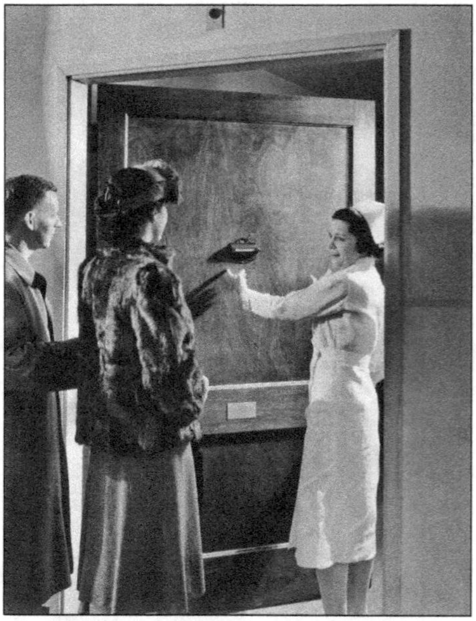

This photograph was part of a capital fundraising campaign to build the West Wing. The building was renamed the Brooks Building in the early 2000s in honor of Braintree resident Harold Brooks, whose trust continues to benefit the hospital years after his death in the 1980s. Many of the hospital's largest gifts are bequests and trusts that allow donors to leave a legacy when an outright gift might be unaffordable.

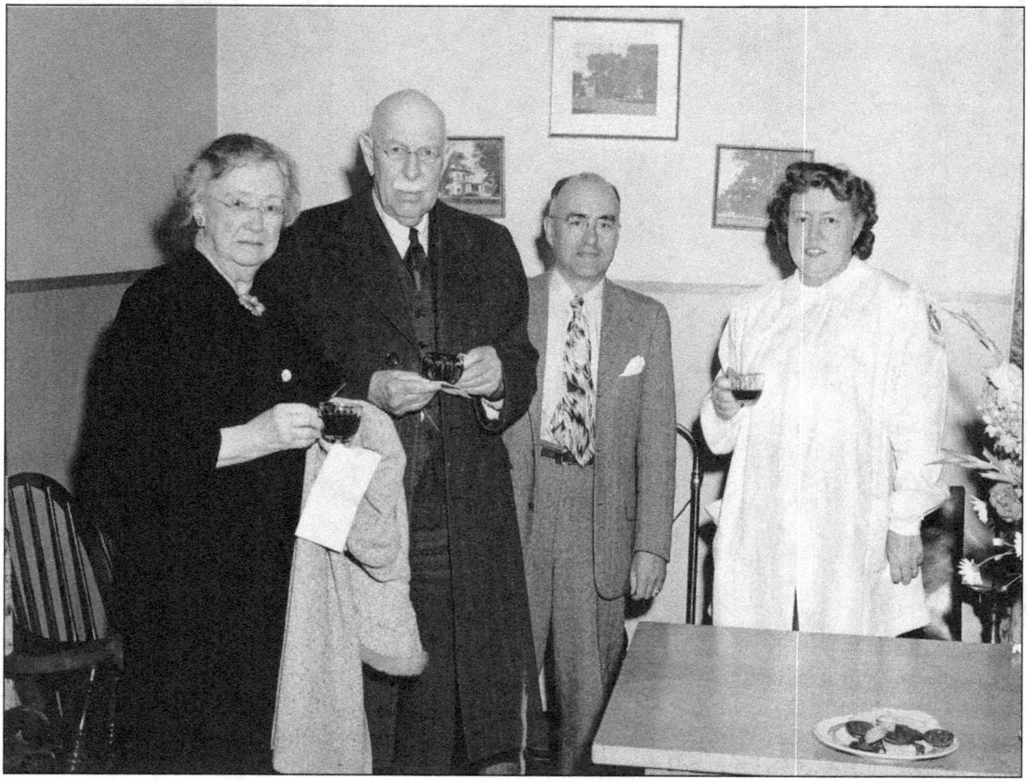

In December 1954, the hospital received $58,000 from Children's Sunlight Hospital, previously part of Frank Lawton's Dreamworld, Scituate. This gift, along with a Ford Foundation grant and community donations, funded improvements to the new Children's Division, including larger rehabilitation areas and a sunny playroom. Reviewing furnishings are, from left to right, Mr. and Mrs. Sumner Chandler, ElectroSwitch president Archie Morrison, and Vernon Marr from Children's Sunlight Hospital.

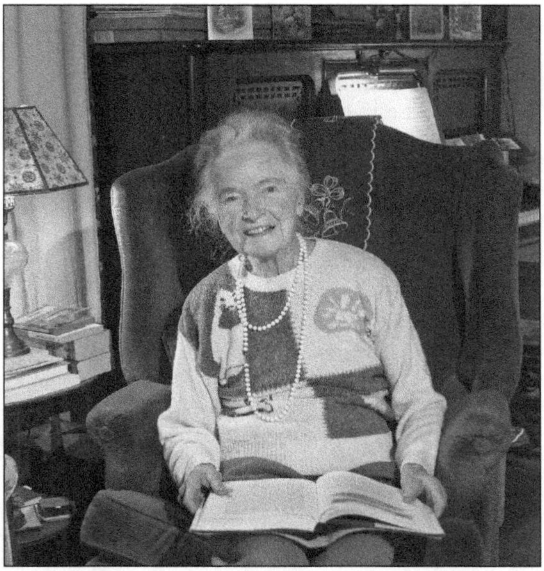

Eleanor Norris donated the 99-acre Norris Reservation in Norwell to the Trustees of the Reservation in memory of her husband. She was a schoolteacher and a philanthropist. By making a planned gift to the hospital, Norris supported care for her neighbors, friends, and the wider community.

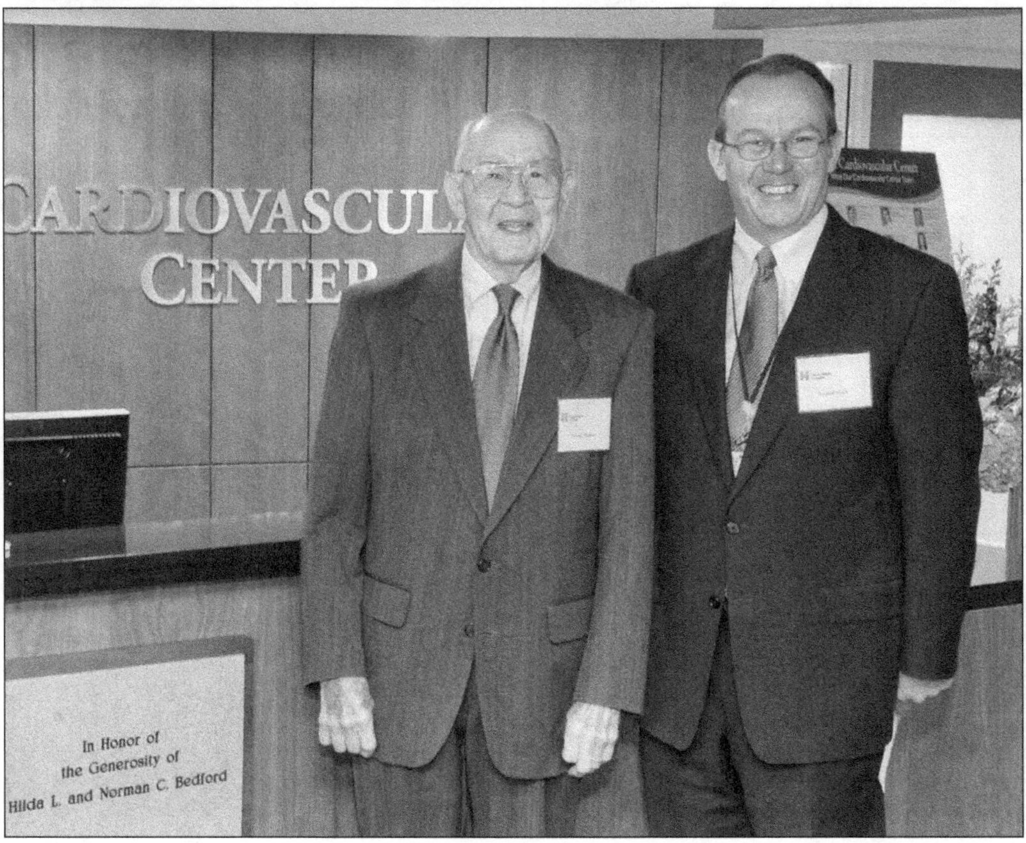
In Honor of
the Generosity of
Hilda L. and Norman C. Bedford

Norman Bedford (left), whose family established the Otis Elevator Company, supported the cardiovascular center, the most comprehensive in the region, after he saw firsthand the center's lifesaving work. From the hospital's earliest days, donors have underwritten the upgrading of equipment and the introduction of new technologies, often when there was no margin in the operating budget. President Richard Aubut (right) welcomes Bedford to the center.

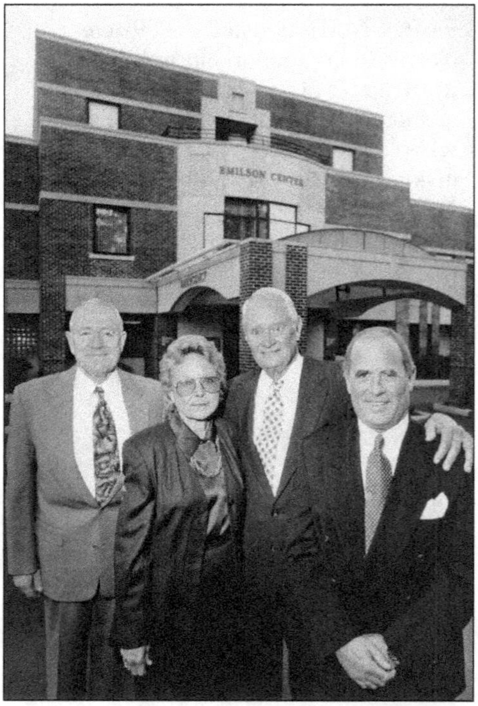

C. Herbert and Paulie Emilson, of North Marshfield, generously support many South Shore charities. Emilson said the hospital improves the lives of more people in the region than any other charity. He and Dr. James Dolphin chaired the capital campaign that funded the expanded maternity and emergency building. Director David Jones (left) and President David Hannan (right) thank the Emilsons in front of the building that bears their name.

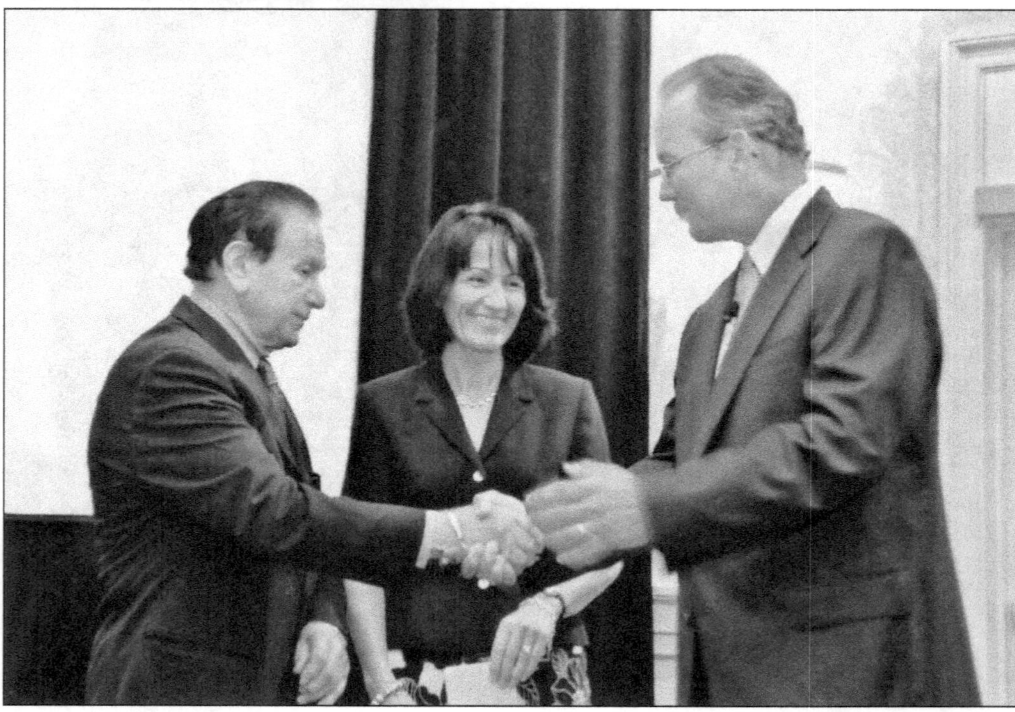

Francis X. Messina, of Braintree, never forgot he was orphaned at an early age. His generosity to the hospital reflected his compassion for families. The F.X. Messina Center houses one of the busiest emergency departments in Massachusetts. The Messina Family Neonatal Intensive Care Unit was the first such Level III unit in a community-based hospital. Hospital president Richard Aubut (right) thanks Messina (left) and his daughter Marissa O'Dwyer.

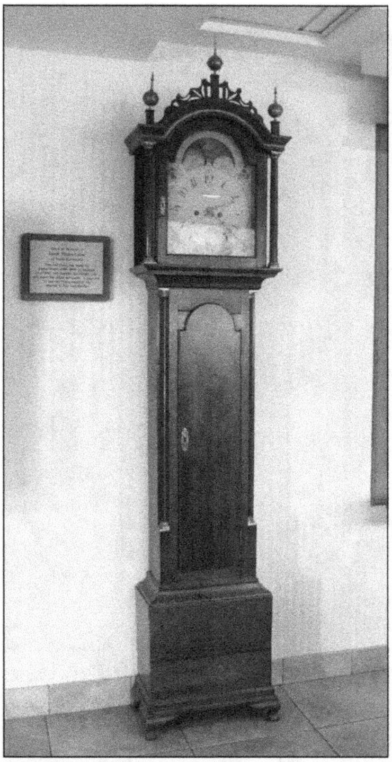

W. Torrey Little, of North Marshfield, donated this tall clock in memory of his wife, Doris Tilden Little. It was made around 1850 by Joshua Wilder, of Hingham, and contains the original case and eight-day brass movement. Little left part of his estate to the hospital, which named the laboratory-materials building in memory of the Littles. (Courtesy of Myrna Walsh.)

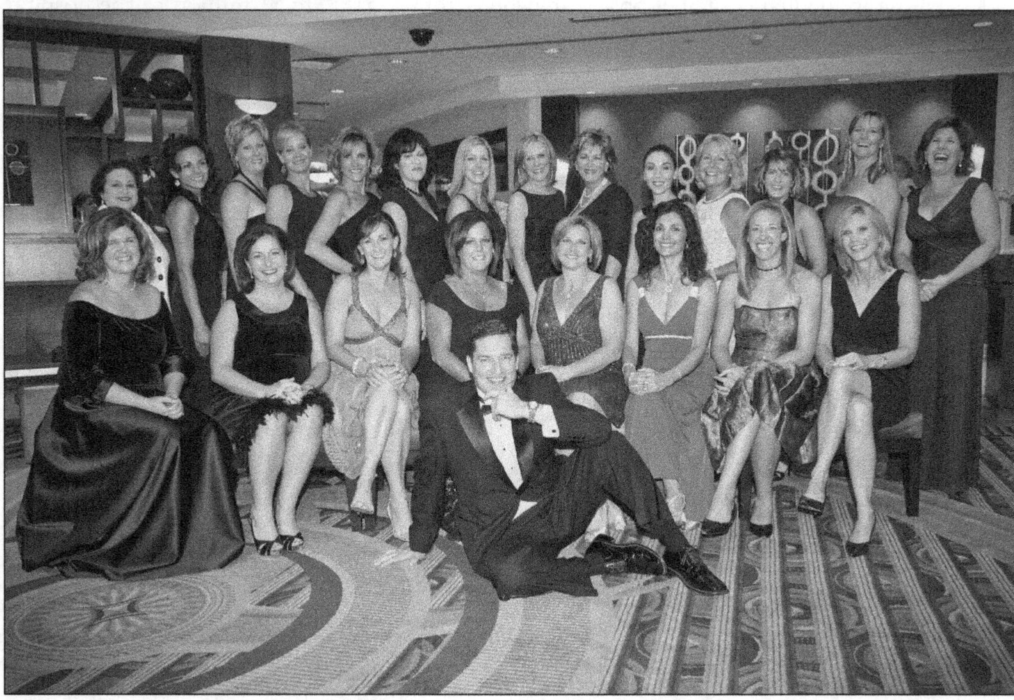

Even during World War II, balls, dinners, and dances were one of the most successful ways to raise funds. Christine Hotarek, of Scituate, and Victoria Hurley, of Cohasset, started the Harvest Moon Ball that became the Moonlight and Miracles Gala, the region's most elegant event. Volunteers like these raised about $2 million for cancer care. The gala and other special events are a cooperative effort between the Foundation and the Friends.

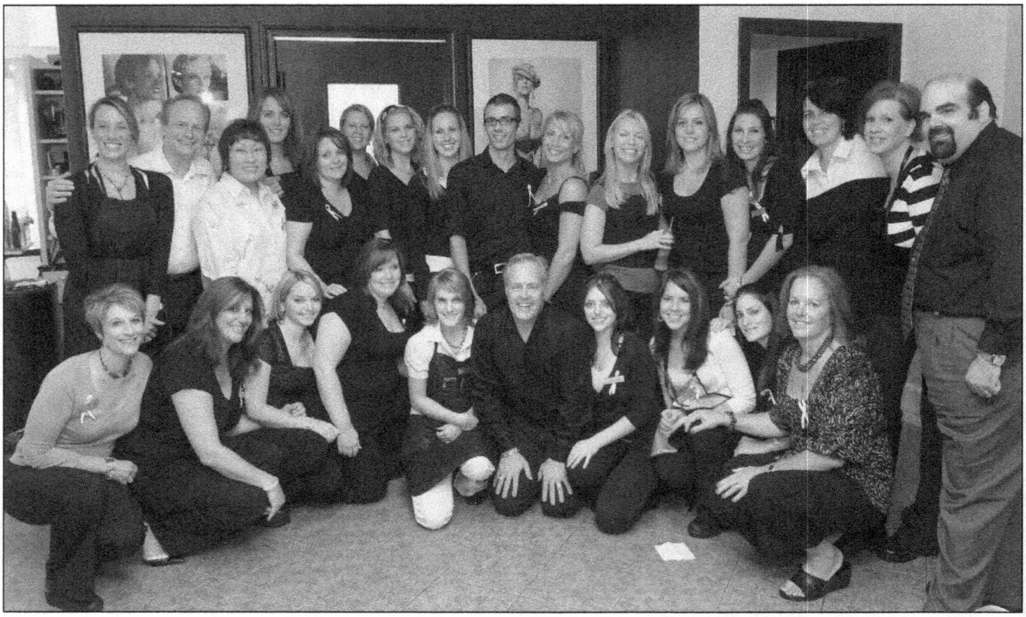

David Honeycutt (standing, second from left), Charles Dudley (kneeling, sixth from left), and the staff of Charles David Salon and Spa work without pay one day a year and donate all proceeds to the hospital's maternity and cancer services. They are members of the Presidents' Circle, business leaders whose individual contributions of anywhere from $25,000 to $1 million to the hospital have totaled $12 million for patient care.

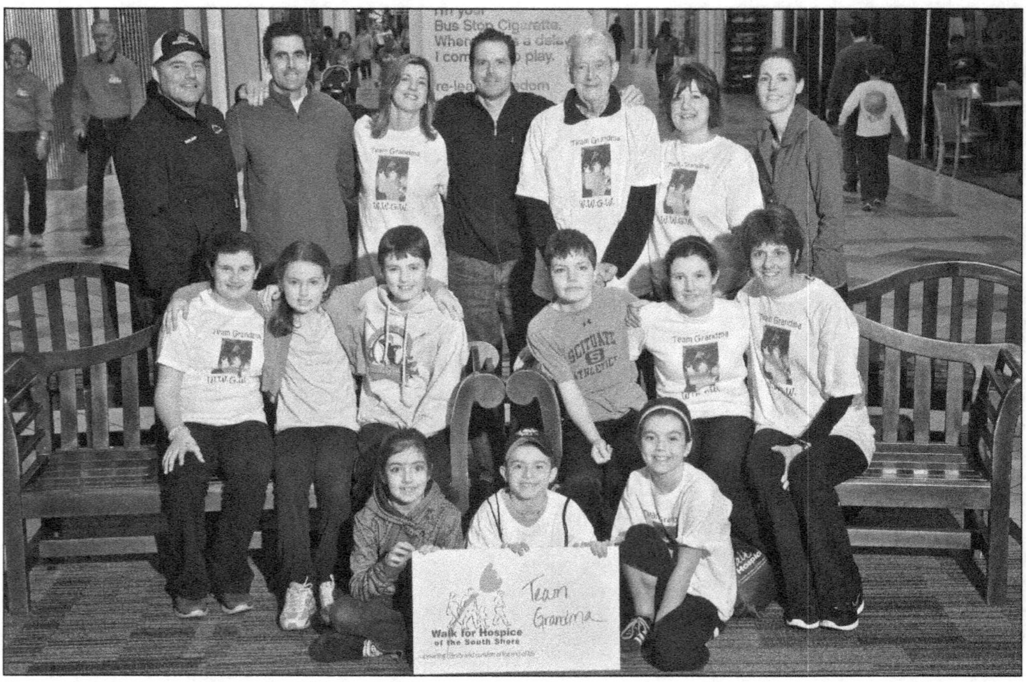

Since it began in 1992, the Walk for Hospice raised almost $2 million for Hospice of the South Shore, the largest hospice in the region. Hospice depends on people and businesses, like Team Grandma, to underwrite care that makes a patient's final time as comfortable as possible. For many families, the fundraiser walk is a memorial and reunion as well as a way to say "thank you."

Nine

Community and Events

Creating a Healthier Community

From the moment Dr. Emerson envisioned the hospital, its most fundamental purpose was to serve the community. It has never wavered.

First, South Shore Hospital benefited the community through clinical programs that addressed southeastern Massachusetts's most prevalent medical conditions—cancer, stroke, heart disease, and trauma.

Second, the hospital has honored its core value of being self-sufficient, especially difficult when Medicare and Medicaid reimbursements were below the cost of providing services to their subscribers. This free and partially funded care costs millions of dollars. The hospital historically paid more into the free-care pool for charity care than other hospitals in the region.

Third, the hospital offered programs to meet the needs of specific groups, such as at-risk youth, the elderly, the impoverished, and those with disabilities and chronic and terminal illnesses. From childbirth classes to bereavement support, hundreds of community programs still dovetail with the founder's goal: the wellbeing of residents.

Even in the 1940s, arguably the hospital's most difficult period, when faced with deficits, overcrowding, lack of resources, and changing leadership, the trustees stayed true to community service.

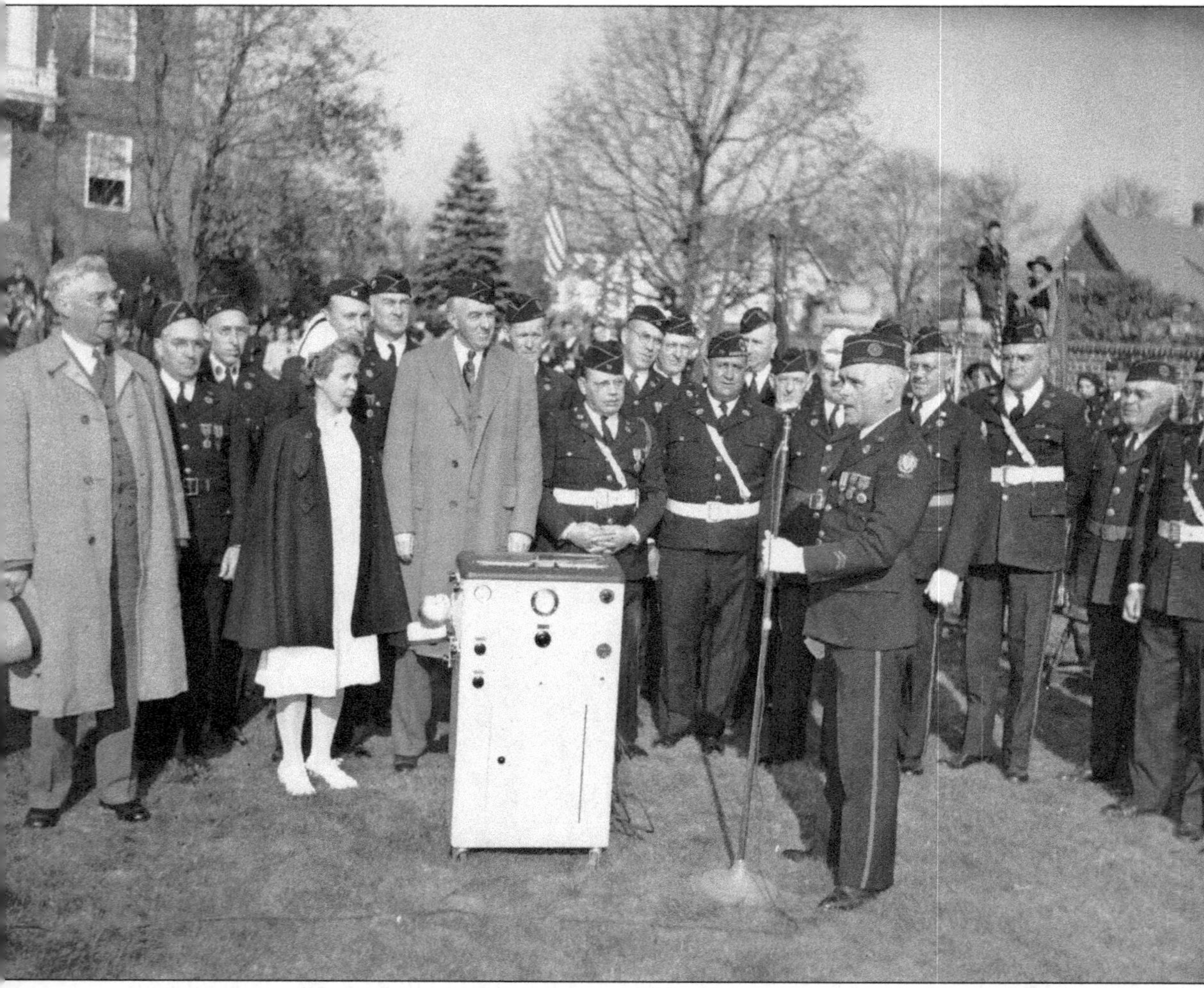

After nearly two decades as hospital superintendent, Eileen Estabrook Oliver was impressive in her flowing nurse's cape, starched cap, and white hose. At Weymouth Town Hall, she accepts an infant incubator from the American Legion. A doll was in the device for the ceremony. In the 1940s, the survival of premature babies improved thanks to incubators.

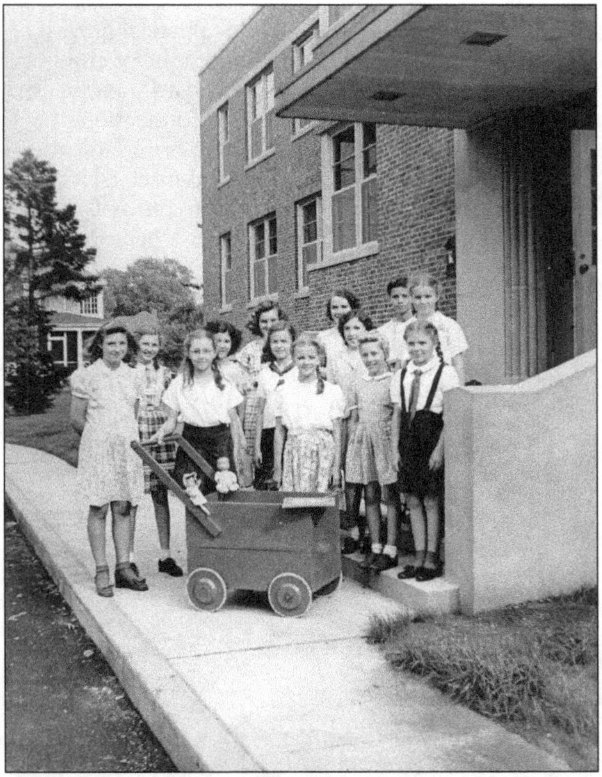

The hospital always garnered support from hundreds of thousands of people of all ages and backgrounds. Among the earliest donors in 1922 were the Orphans Hope Lodge A.F. and A.M., the Loggia Giuseppe Verde, Lodge No. 28, Sons of Italy, the Christian Endeavor Society of North Weymouth, the North Weymouth Home Economics Club, and the Abigail Adams Rebekan Lodge. Weymouth children have generously supported the hospital, often with homegrown vegetables and flowers, books, and toys. In the photograph at left, children deliver toys for pediatric patients in 1941. Below, Girl Scouts from Troop 3532 follow that tradition 50 years later by donating books to hospitalized youngsters. The Friends' Leaders Involving New Kinds of Support (LINKS) group designated pediatric services as the beneficiary of its special events.

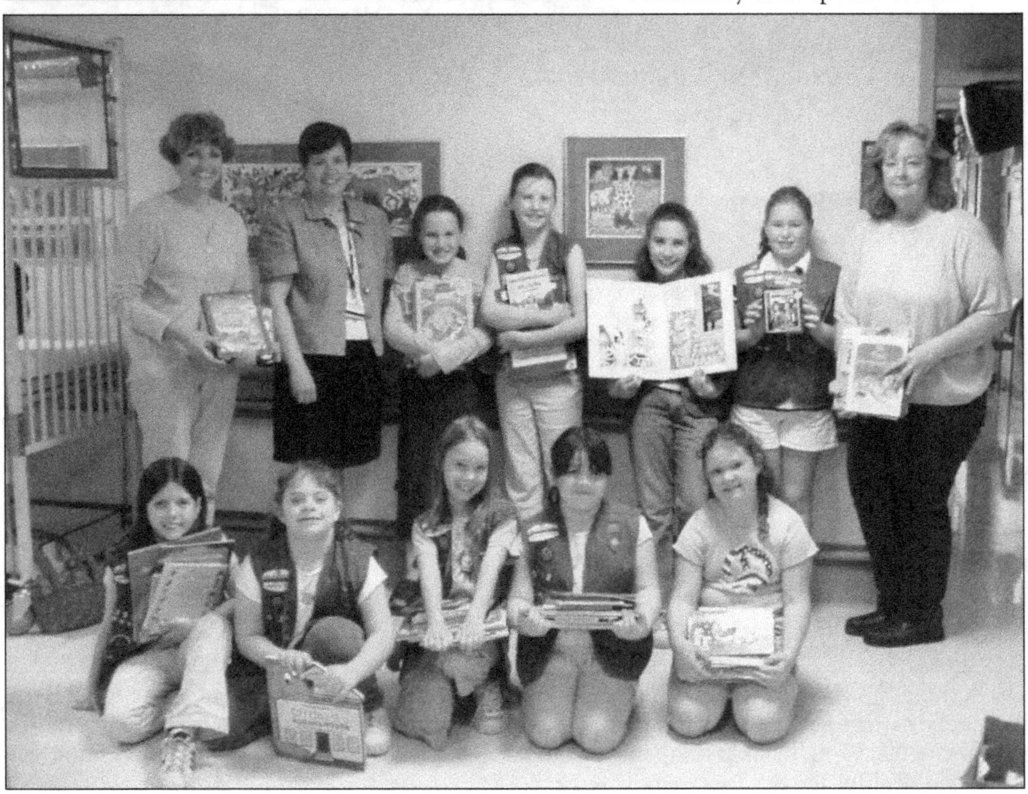

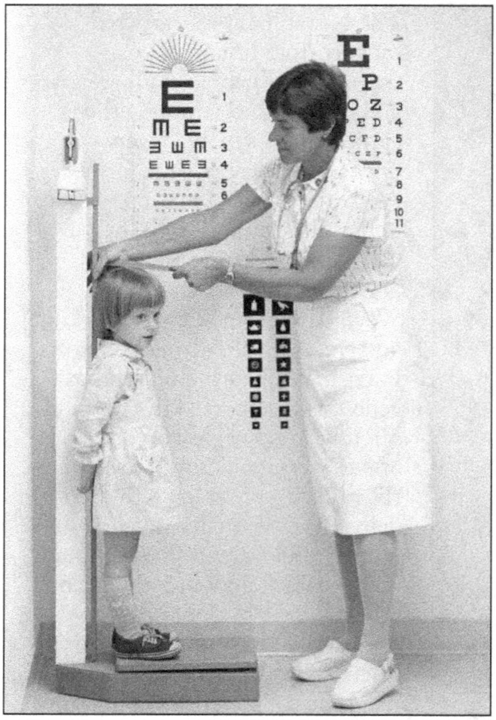

Whether checking a child's physical growth or mental well being, the hospital helps children make good decisions to safeguard their health. Through the Youth Health Connection, it has a unique partnership that brings together students, parents, teachers, counselors, and hospital and VNA staff to prevent adolescent suicide and high-risk behavior.

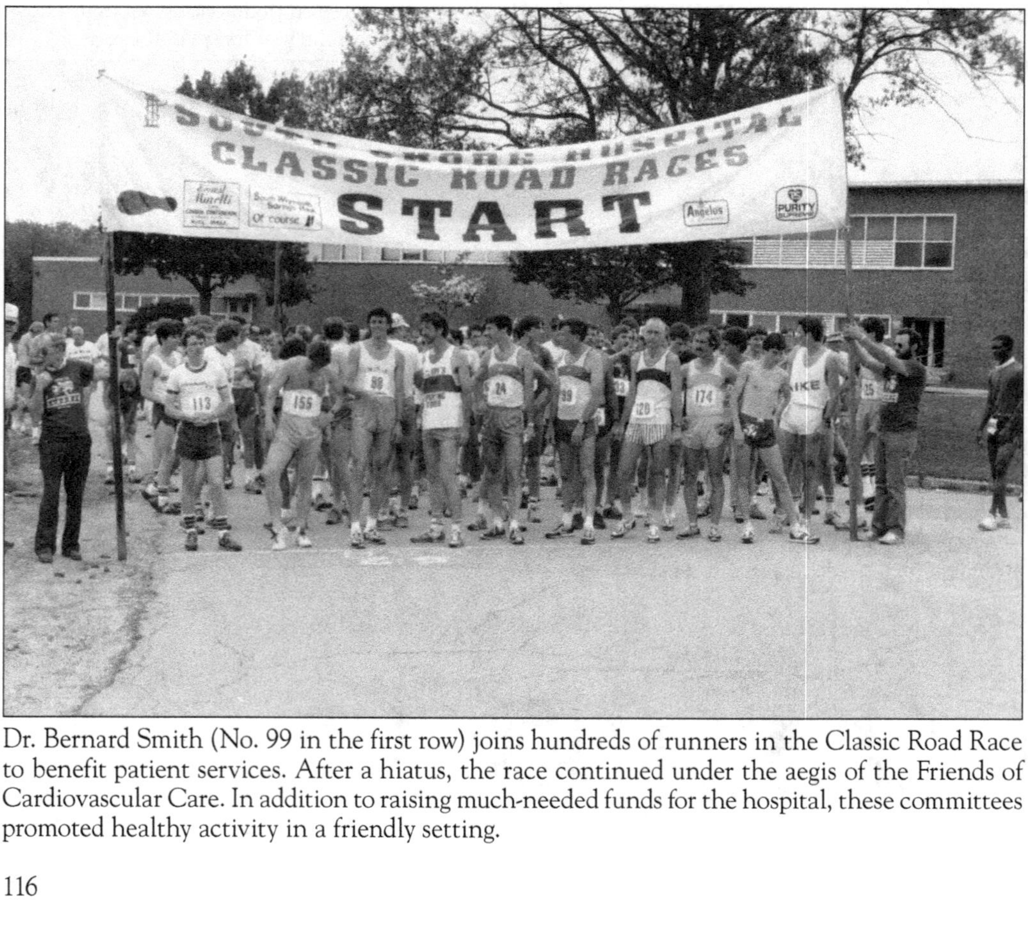

Dr. Bernard Smith (No. 99 in the first row) joins hundreds of runners in the Classic Road Race to benefit patient services. After a hiatus, the race continued under the aegis of the Friends of Cardiovascular Care. In addition to raising much-needed funds for the hospital, these committees promoted healthy activity in a friendly setting.

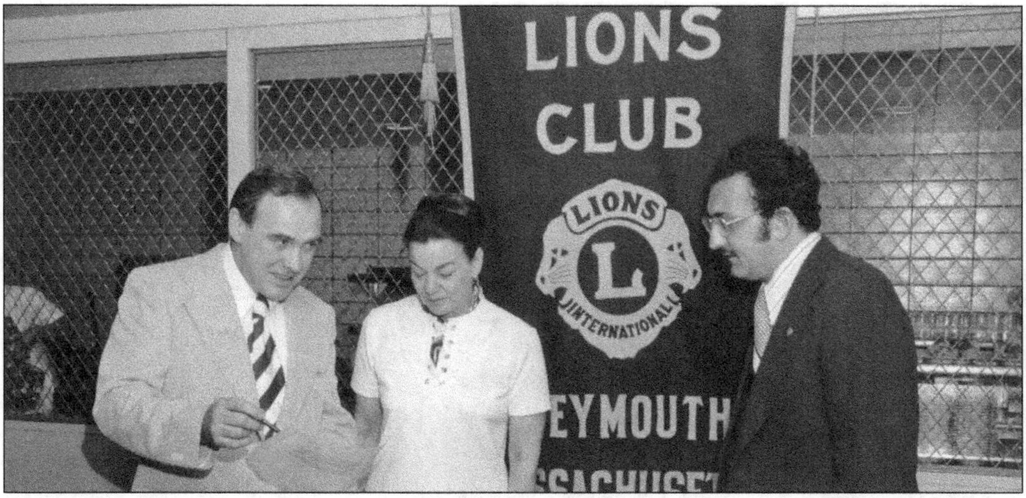

Support from community organizations, like the Lions, Rotary, and Kiwanis, dates back to 1922. Here, unidentified members of the Weymouth Lions Club make a donation to Joan Roche. The hospital and its home-care division continued to be the charities of choice with more than $15 million donated annually through the South Shore Hospital Charitable Foundation, formerly South Shore Health and Educational Foundation.

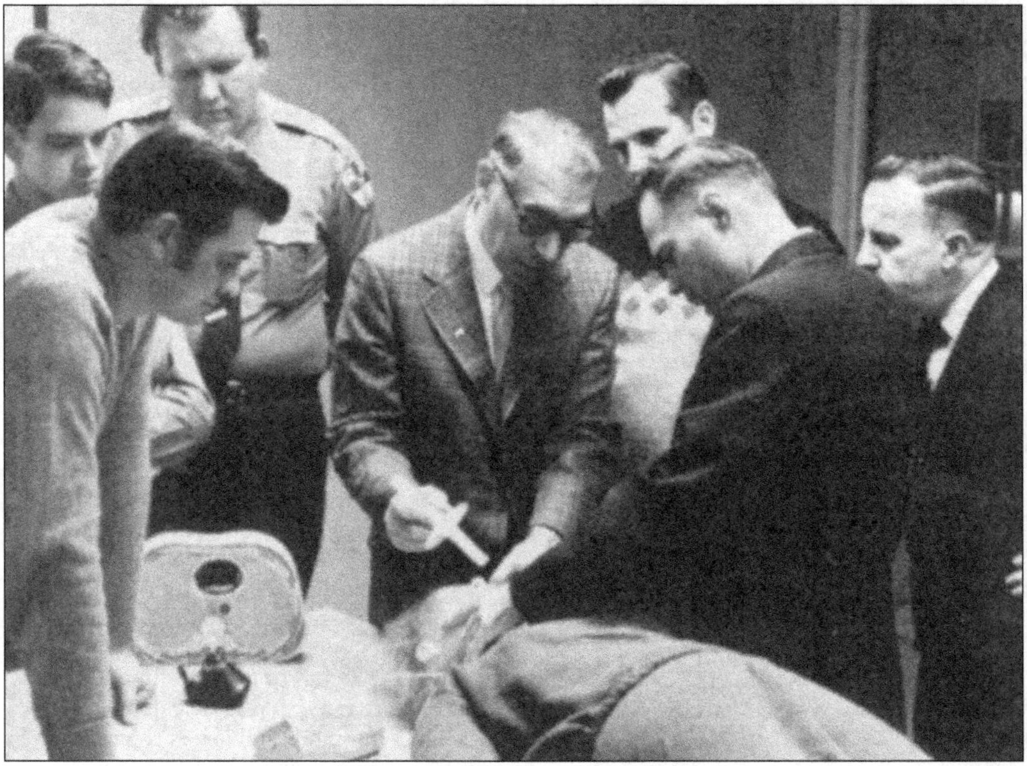
Dr. Herman Beal (center) demonstrates CPR at a community program, one of many offered at little or no fee. These continue to be tailored to a variety of conditions, including Parkinson's, osteoporosis, obstructed lung disease, and bereavement. They generate little or no margin and would likely be discontinued if the hospital were not a charity and if its leaders made decisions on a purely financial basis.

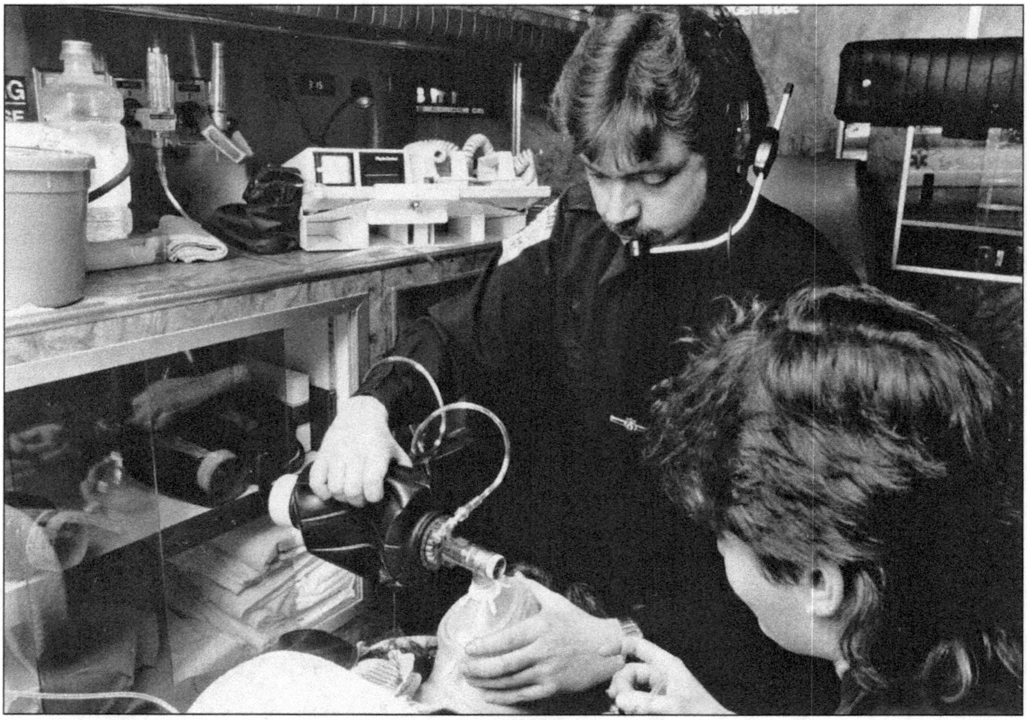

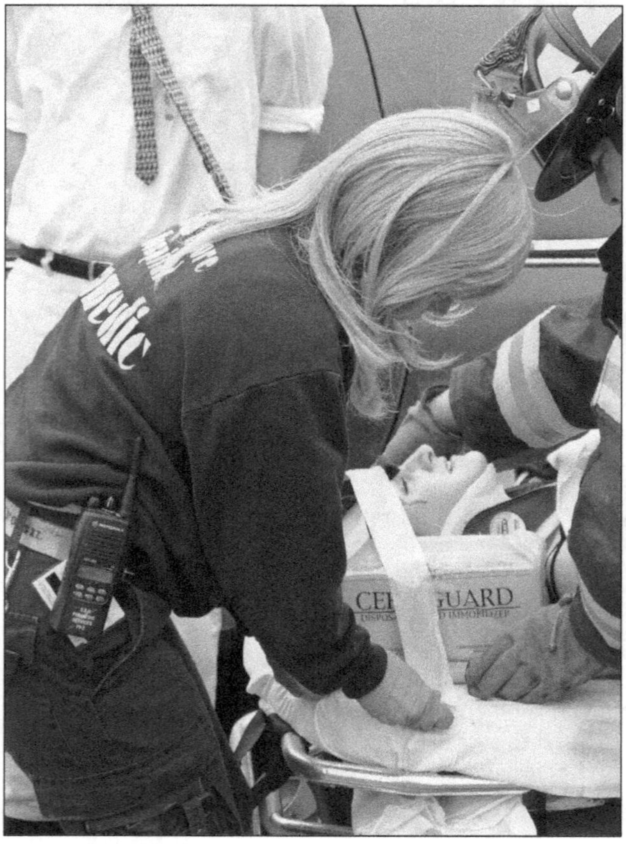

For many towns on the South Shore, employing full-time paramedics was expensive. South Shore Hospital offered the services of full-time paramedics who meet the towns' ambulances at accidents and other emergencies and provide immediate assistance when minutes count. The hospital also conducted regular disaster drills with the towns and maintained a decontamination facility for chemical or nuclear disasters. The hospital participated in demonstrations of mock automobile crashes to show high school students the dangers of drinking and driving. Staff was at the forefront of encouraging and training coaches to identify concussions. To treat serious accidents, the hospital established the region's first designated trauma center.

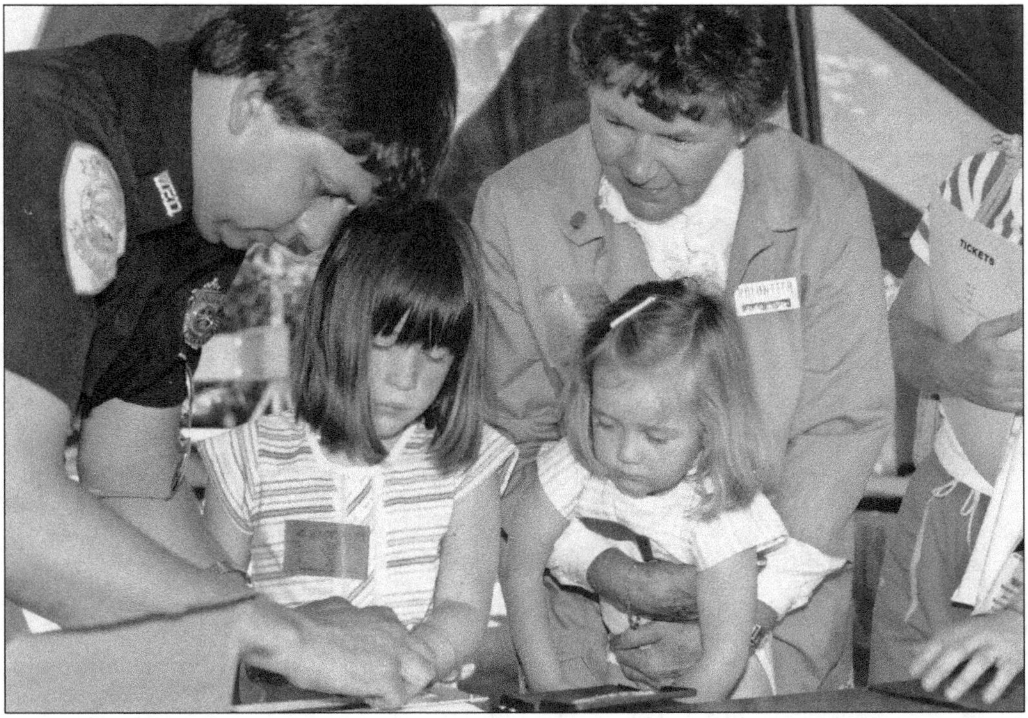

A Weymouth police officer fingerprints youngsters as part of a national program to identify lost or abducted children. The hospital often coordinated with local towns to offer health and safety clinics and fairs. One of the most comprehensive programs involved Weymouth and the hospital working to reduce cardiovascular disease through a commonwealth Mass in Motion grant.

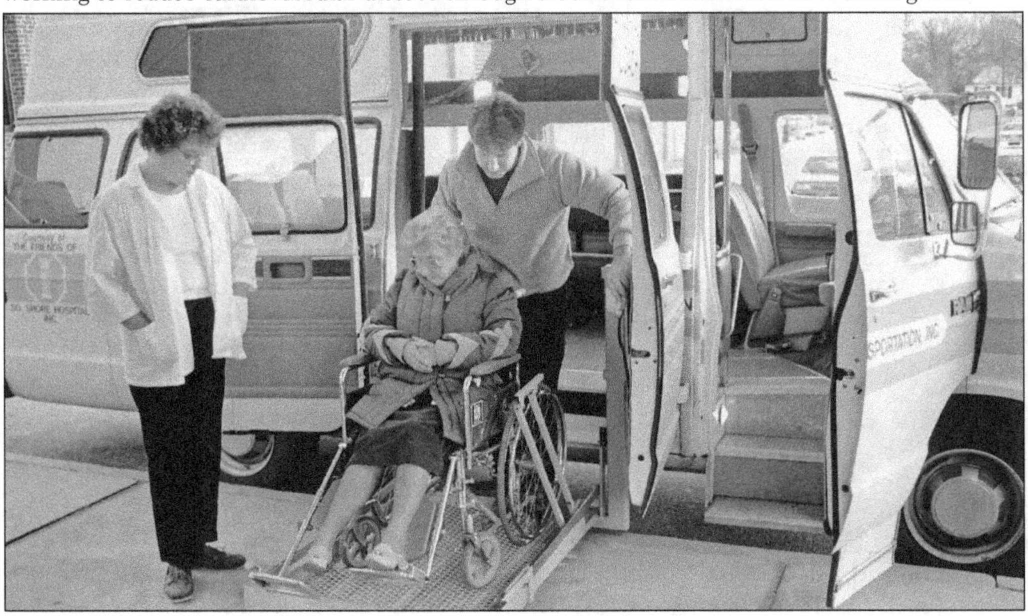

A woman is assisted to a doctor's appointment in 1990 via a van donated by the Friends. For elders who no longer can drive or those without automobiles, this van literally can be a lifesaver. Over the years, the hospital invested millions in community programs that help residents improve their lifestyles and maintain their health.

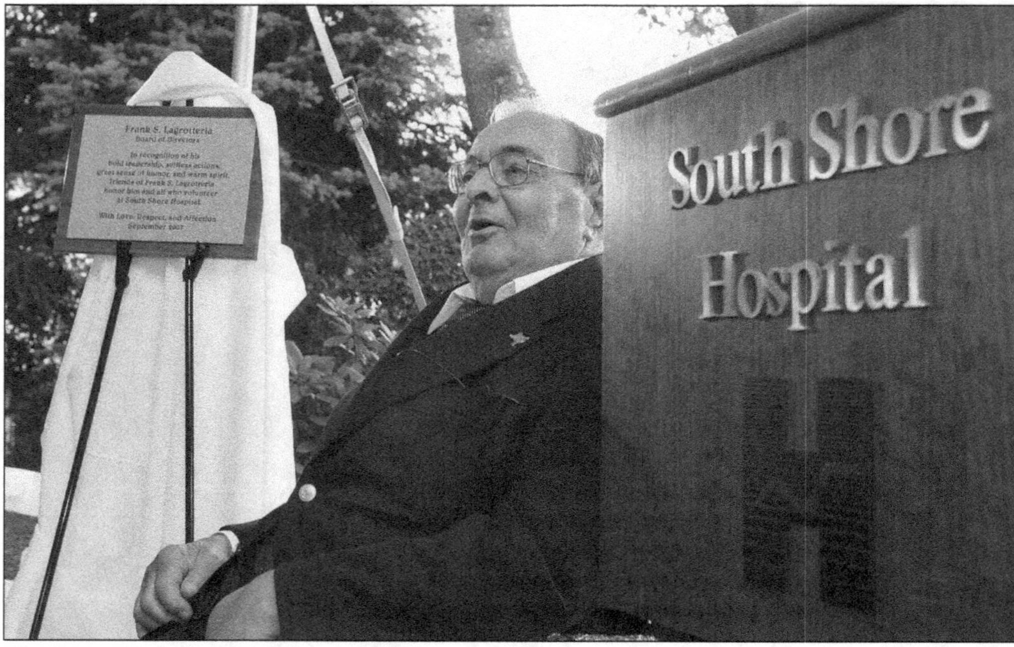

The hospital is owned by the community, not shareholders, who help define the communities' needs. Former board member and overseer Frank Lagrotteria is honored "with love, respect and affection, in recognition of his bold leadership, selfless actions, great sense of humor and warm spirit." He was also Weymouth's town engineer and director of public works. The public works headquarters at 120 Winter Street is named in his honor.

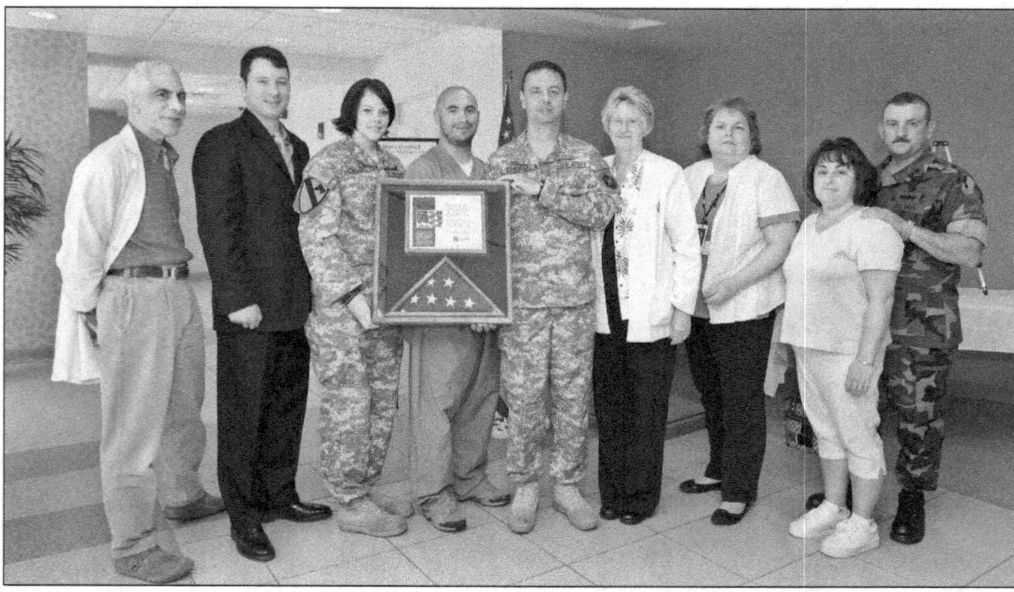

Hospital staff served America. In World War II, 29 nurses and 18 of the hospital's 28 physicians enlisted, including its sole roentgenologist. Shown 60 years later, colleagues who served or had family serving are, from left to right, Dr. Robert Gore, William Carron, Amanda Cataldo, Nicolas Bruce, Paul and Jeanne Zaborski, Donna Leadbetter, and Lisa and Keith Jermyn. They are presenting a flag flown at the 399th Combat Support Hospital at an American forward operating base in Iraq.

Ten

In the Spotlight

Visits by the Powerful and Famous

As South Shore Hospital grew in stature, celebrities from sports, entertainment, and politics were drawn to its doors. When celebrities visit patients, those moments of cheer and encouragement provide memories that may last a lifetime. They also add sparkle to fundraising events.

The visits with leaders in the political world have a more serious purpose. South Shore Hospital is on the frontline of delivering health care and offers lawmakers a perspective that is valuable in deciding state and national policy. As a pioneer in introducing services that once would have been available only at academic medical centers, the hospital operates efficiently while providing quality care.

With its huge constituencies of patients and their families, 3,800 employees, 880 physicians, and hundreds of thousands of donors, the hospital speaks with authority.

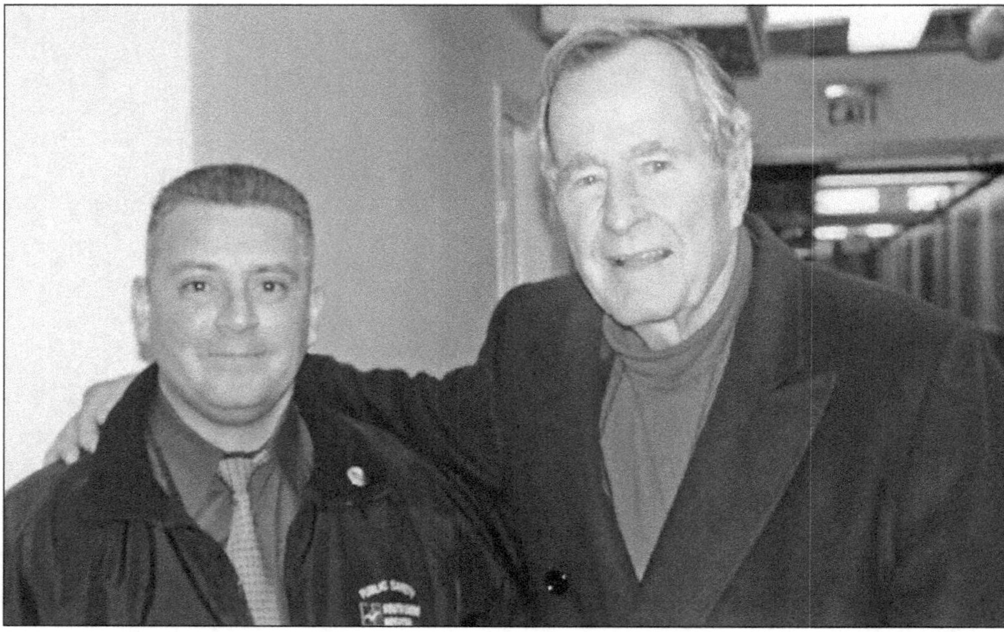

On a private visit, Pres. George H.W. Bush (right) graciously stopped to speak with staff and pose for a candid photograph with Nelson Lugo. The hospital's security worked closely with the Secret Service, which protects American presidents even when retired. Unless they waive privacy, patients are assured that all private information remains strictly confidential, whether they are rock stars or more private citizens.

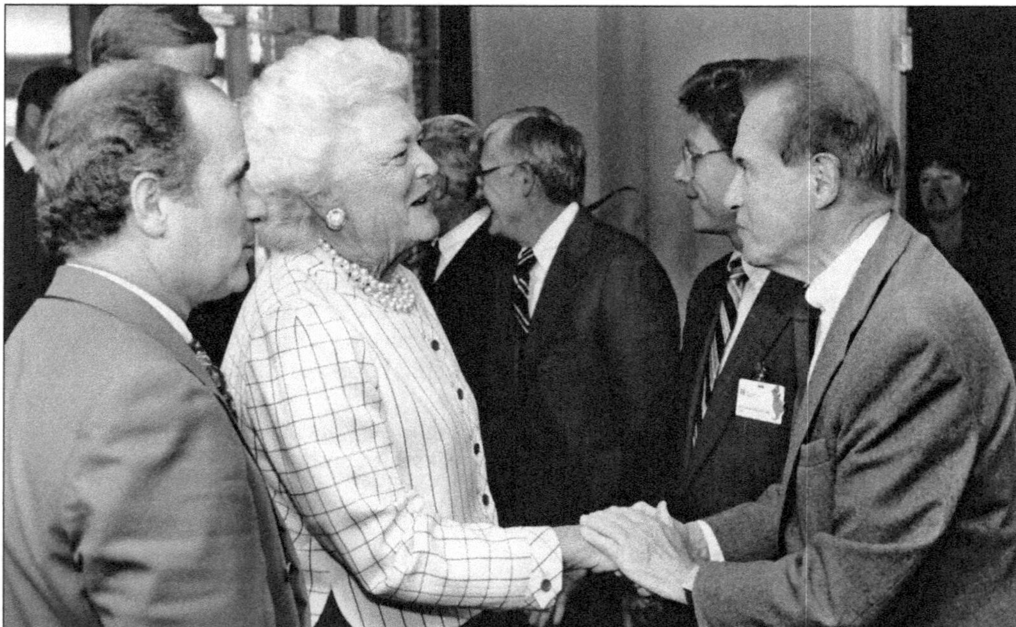

First Lady Barbara Bush was interested in care for infants, especially the frailest in the neonatal intensive care unit, one of the first in a community hospital in the commonwealth. A solarium in the hospital was named in her honor. Hospital president David Hannan (left) introduces Director Henry Hoffman (right) to the first lady.

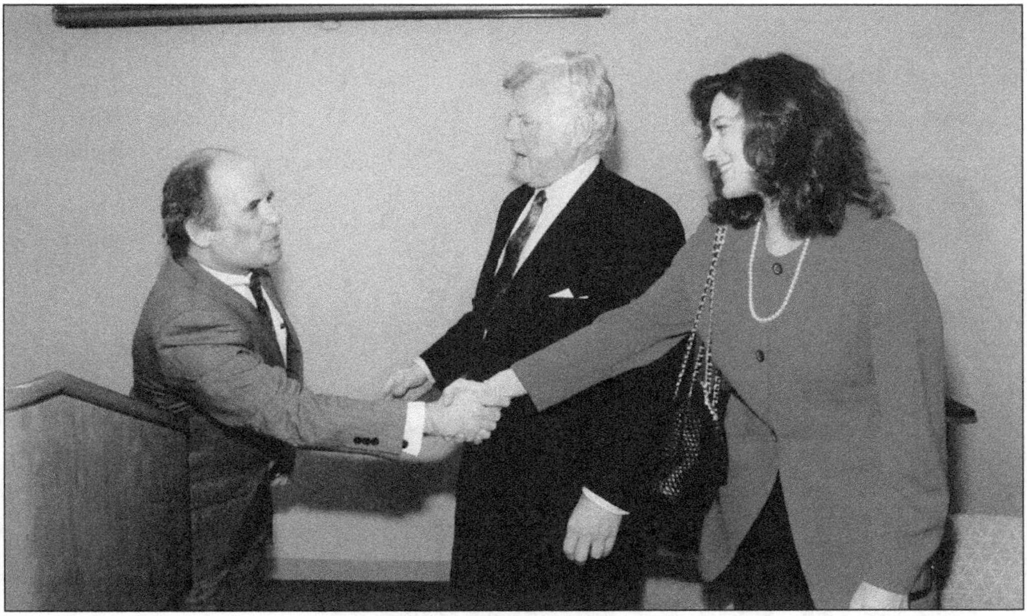

US senator Edward Kennedy (center) visited the hospital many times throughout his long career. As the senate's leading proponent of health care reform, he listened to the opinions of the hospital leaders and staff, but did not live to see the reforms passed. Hospital president David Hannan greets Senator Kennedy and his wife, Victoria.

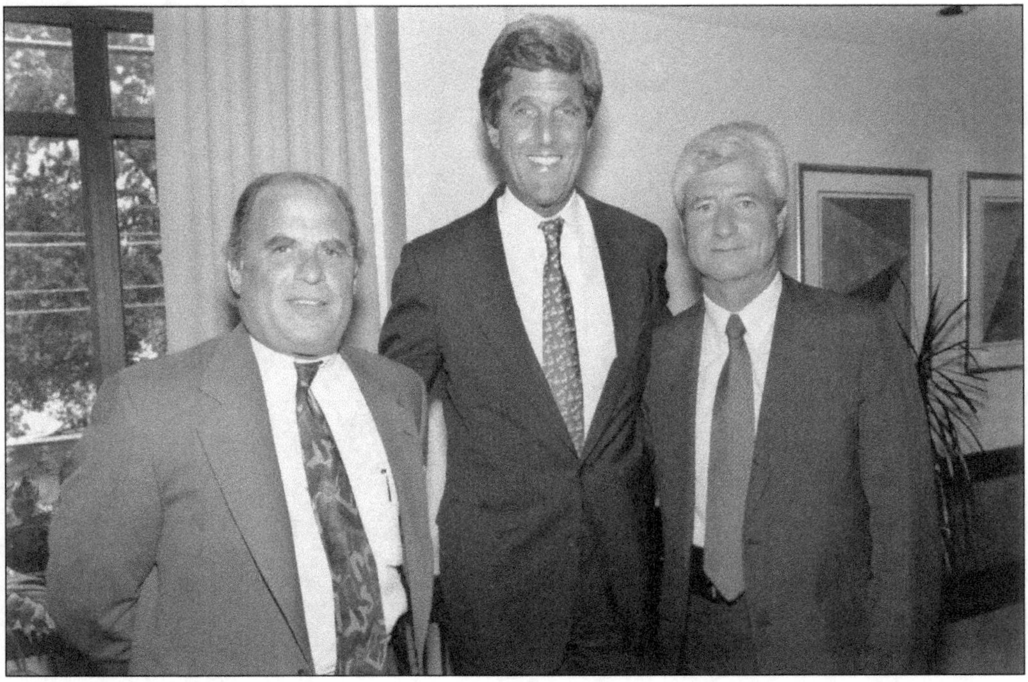

In 1994, US senator John Kerry (center), later Democratic candidate for president, meets with hospital president David Hannan (left) and medical staff president Charles Gaughan to learn how the hospital provides care that is consistently recognized as among the best in the country. Candidates often visited the hospital to meet with its leaders and to attend "town meetings" with physicians and employees.

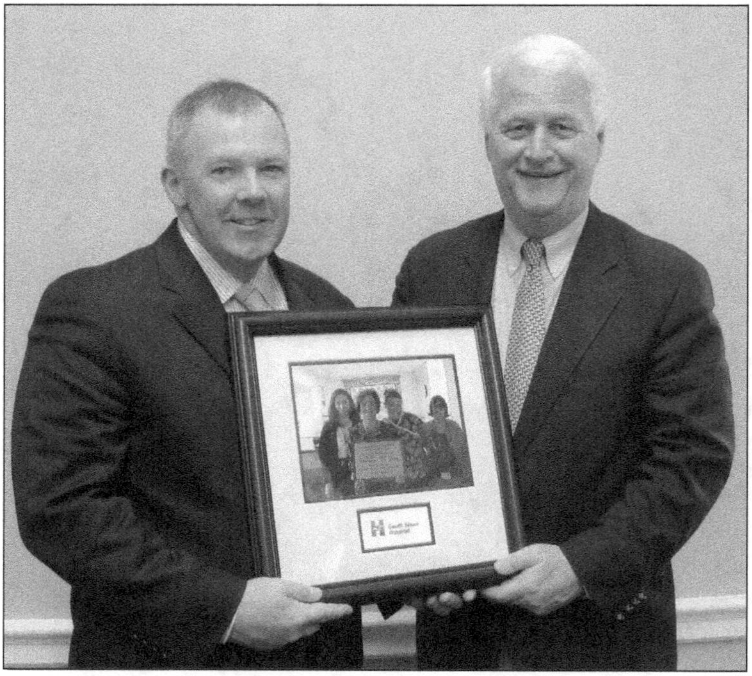

Robert Frazer (left), president of South Coastal Bank and a member of the hospital's Presidents' Circle, thanks US representative William Delahunt, who obtained funding for the hospital's neonatal intensive care unit. He also helped secure funding for CT scanners. This core equipment in the hospital's stroke center assists neurologists in diagnosing strokes faster and more accurately.

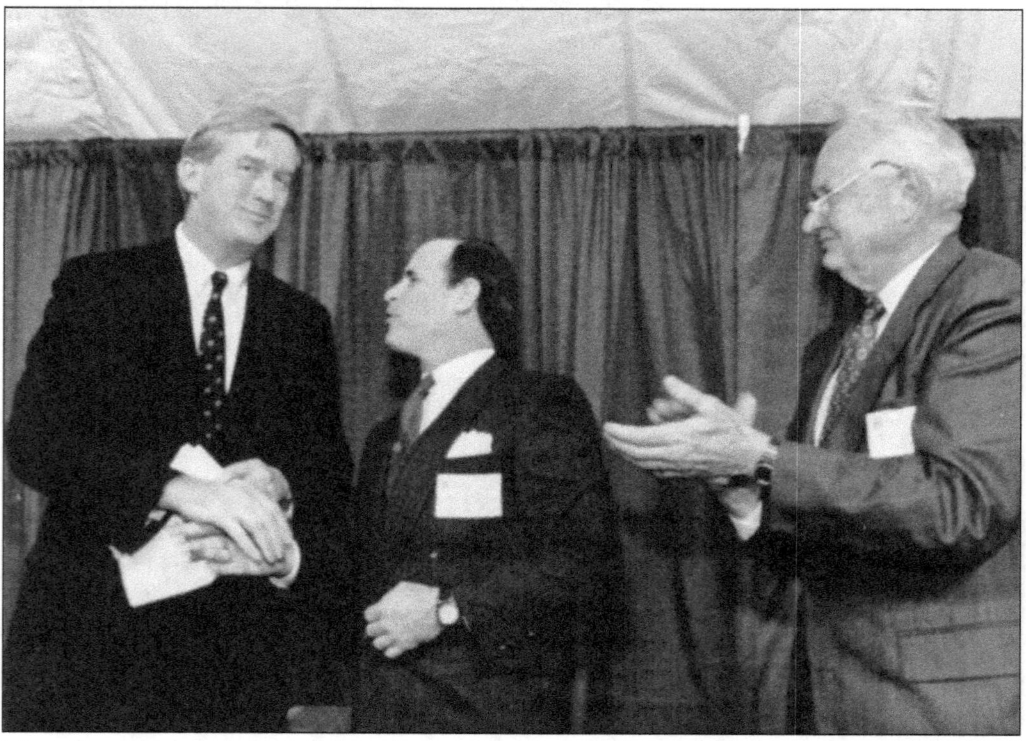

More than 800 people heard Massachusetts governor William Weld speak at the new building dedication ceremony in 1991. Governor Weld (left) is thanked by hospital president David Hannan (center) and C. Herbert Emilson, chairman of the building's fundraising committee. When Weld's lieutenant governor Paul Cellucci was elected governor, he too visited the hospital several times, as did Govs. Jane Swift, Mitt Romney, and Deval Patrick.

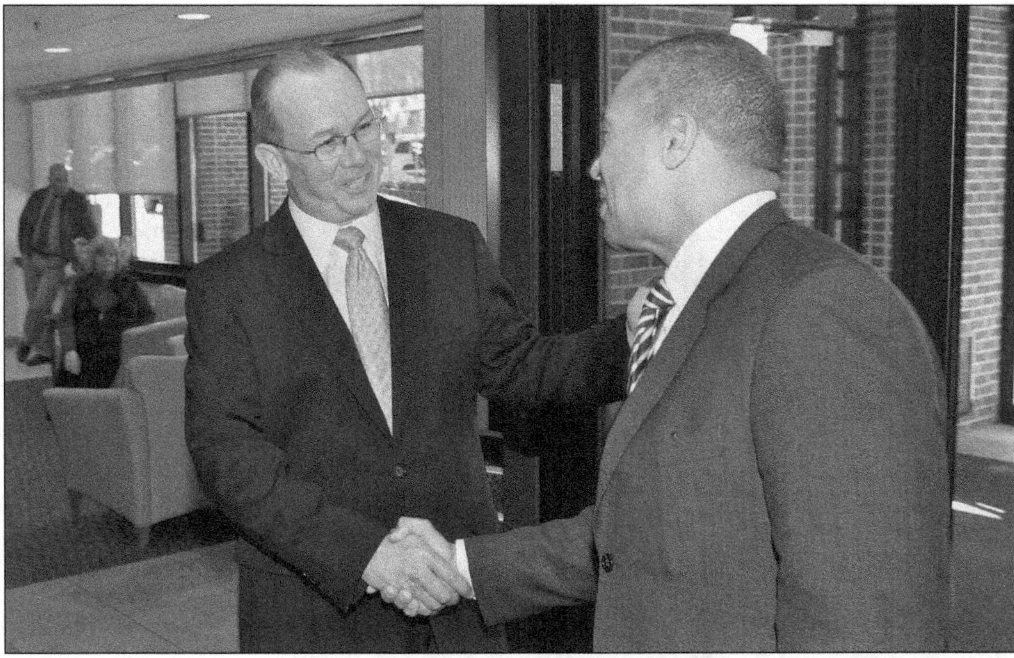

Massachusetts governor Deval Patrick visited the hospital when he announced the first anniversary status of the commonwealth's health care plan. He noted that he chose South Shore Hospital because it reduced costs while improving quality of healthcare. President Richard Aubut (left) hosts Patrick on a hospital tour and a session with physicians.

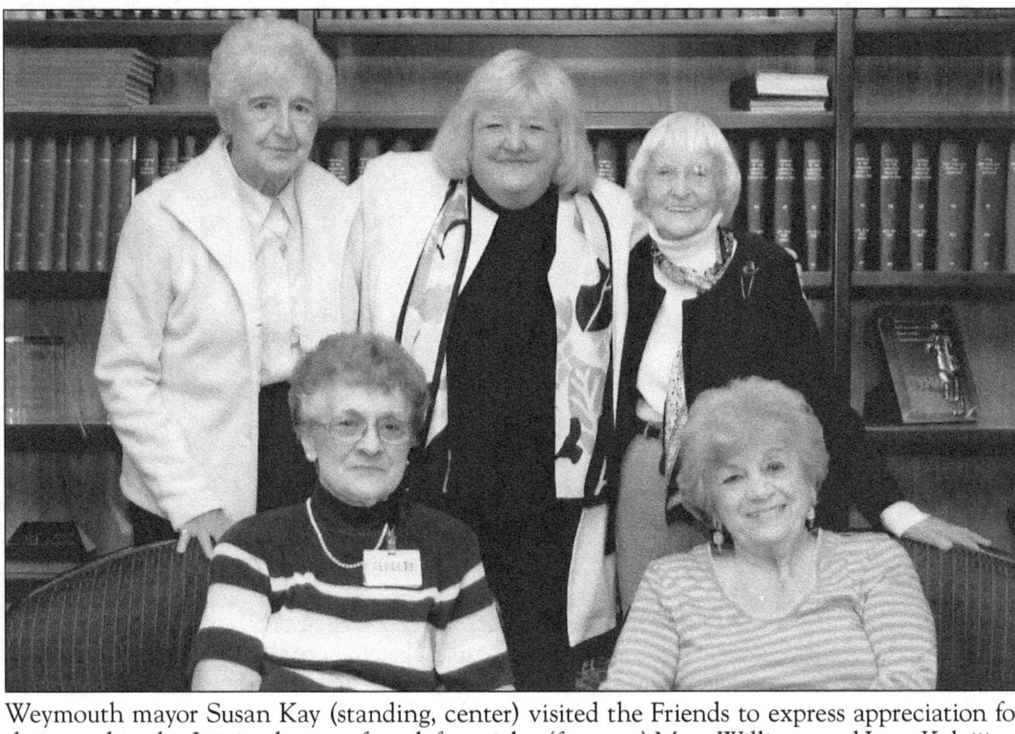

Weymouth mayor Susan Kay (standing, center) visited the Friends to express appreciation for their good works. Joining her are, from left to right, (first row) Mary Williams and Lucy Kalaijian; (second row) Claire Plourde and Diane Sheehan, all from Weymouth.

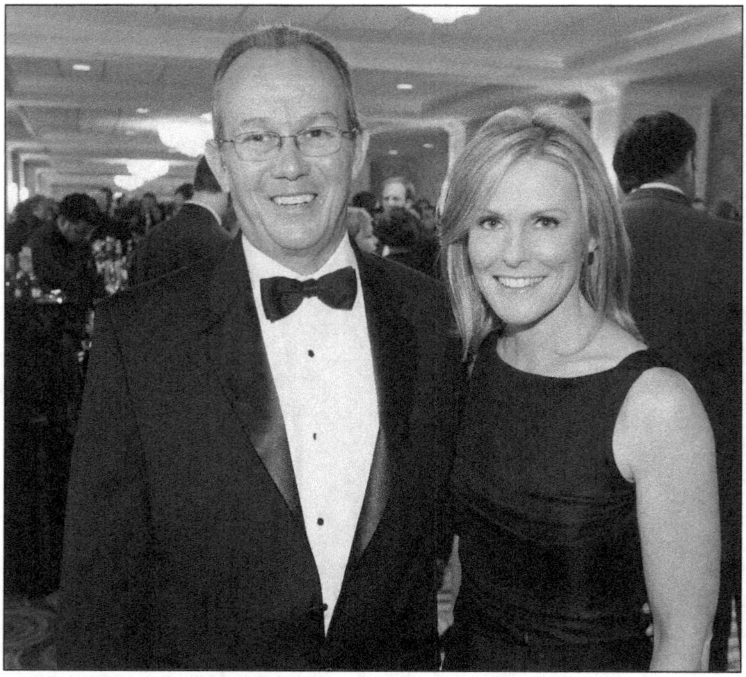

President Richard Aubut welcomes WBZ news anchor Lisa Hughes as mistress of ceremonies at the Friends' Moonlight and Miracles Gala. The premiere gala raised $2 million for cancer care over time. The hospital's cancer programs, in affiliation with Brigham and Women's Hospital and Dana-Farber Cancer Institute, bring oncology experts, advanced diagnostic imaging, and clinical trials closer to home for regional residents.

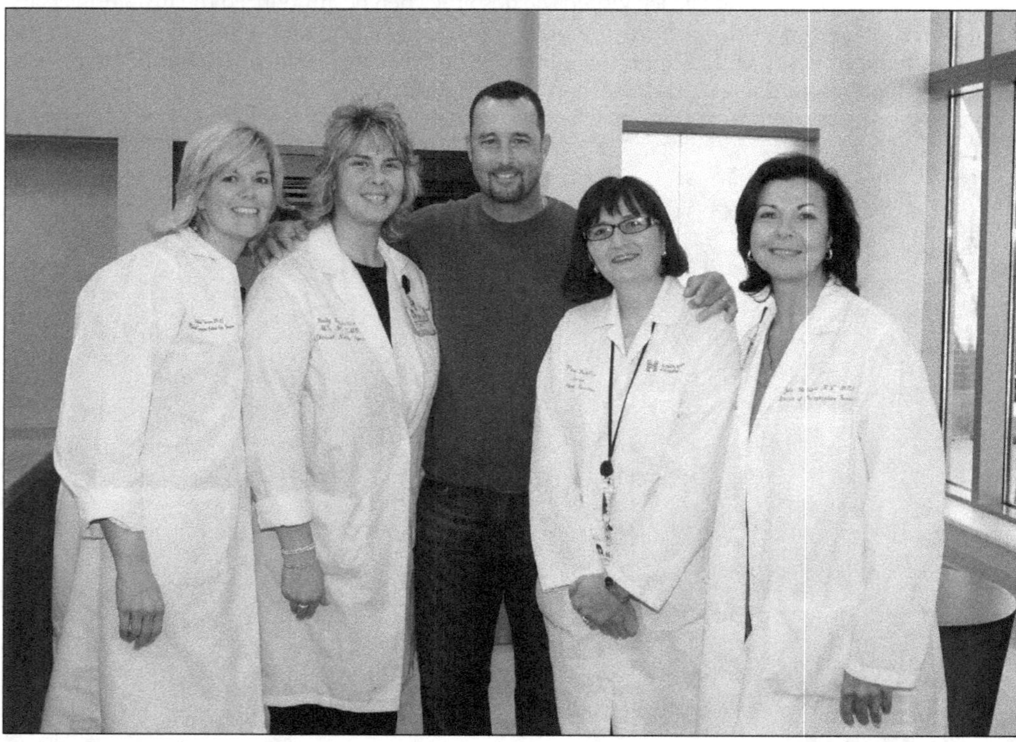

Red Sox pitcher Tim Wakefield (center) tours the hospital before he and his wife accept honorary chairmanships of the Moonlight and Miracles Gala. A local resident, he is an avid hospital supporter, even more so after visiting patients. Here he greets, from left to right, Charlene Freccero (nurse manager), Kelly Fitzpatrick (clinical nurse specialist), Paula Beaulieu (emergency department director), and Julie McIntyre (perioperative director).

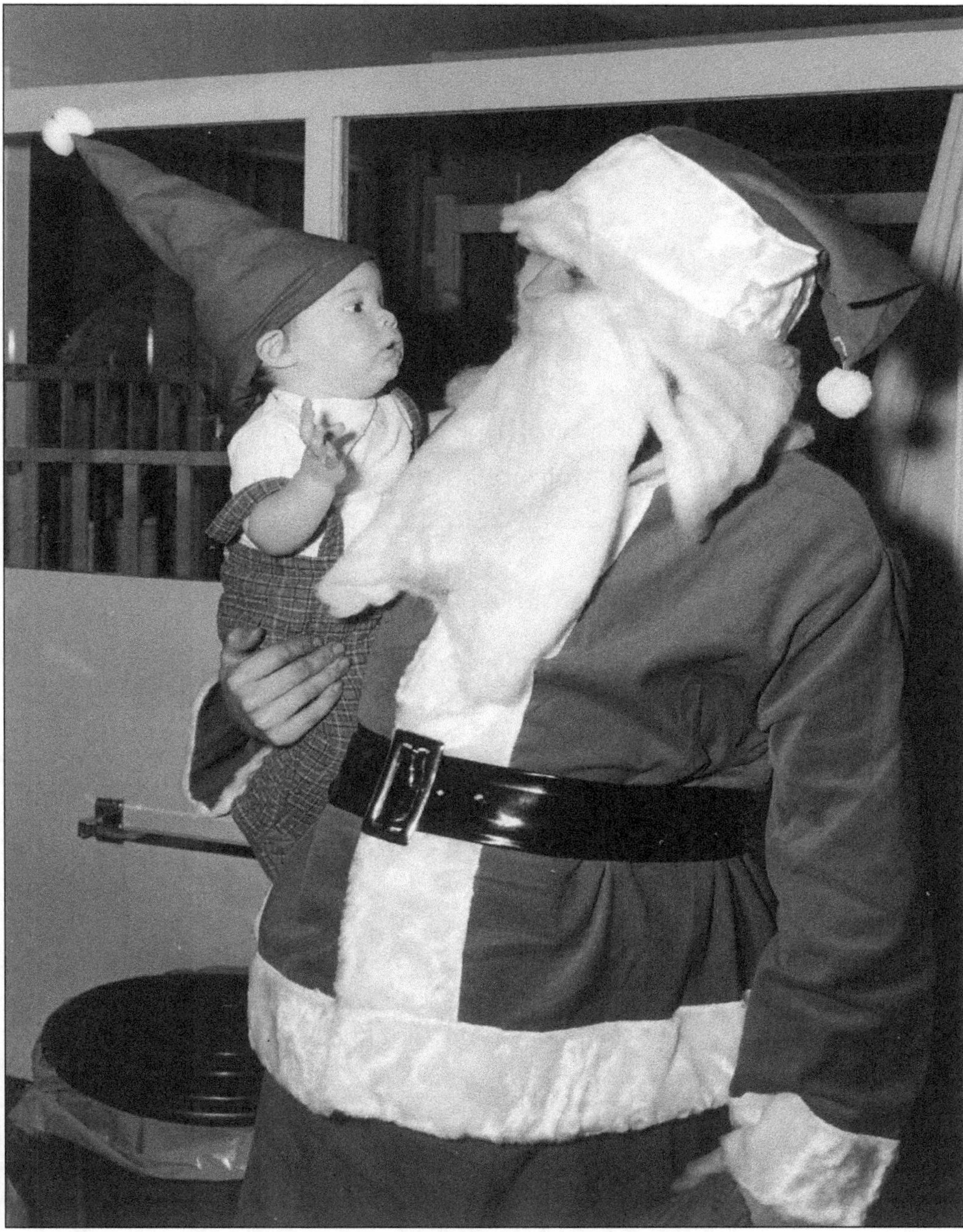

Comforting patients and their families is as much a part of the hospital mission as healing. Here is one celebrity who has changed little over the years. Members of the Friends and volunteers dress as Santa and sing carols in the pediatric units. Often, local school children donate books or toys, and the nurses decorate the rooms and hallways. The baby in this 1950s photograph may have later had her children at South Shore Hospital, and they likely returned to have their children. The hospital's legacy is of one generation investing in care for the next. As with all great institutions, past is prologue to the future. Written in 1954, board president Roy W. Lawson's words still ring true: "As with any vibrant organization which is operating successfully, we have new lines of endeavor to follow and new goals to be reached. There is much unfinished business before us."

www.ingramcontent.com/pod-product-compliance
Lightning Source LLC
LaVergne TN
LVHW081933200926
848484LV00009B/2417
* 9 7 8 1 5 3 1 6 5 0 8 3 4 *